# If You Give A Boy A Garden

Danielle M. Jackson

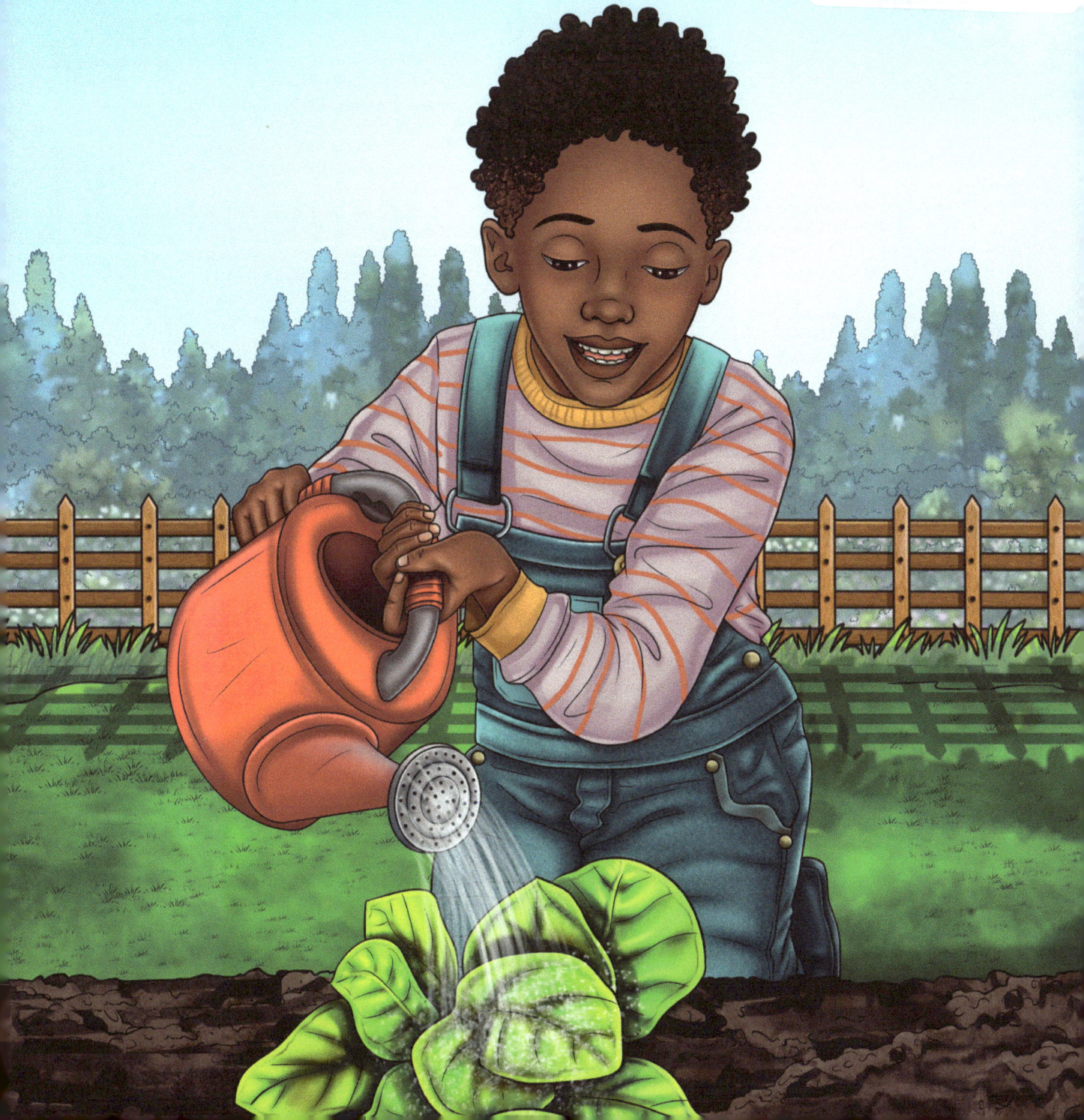

If you give a boy a garden, he'll ask you to teach him how to grow food.

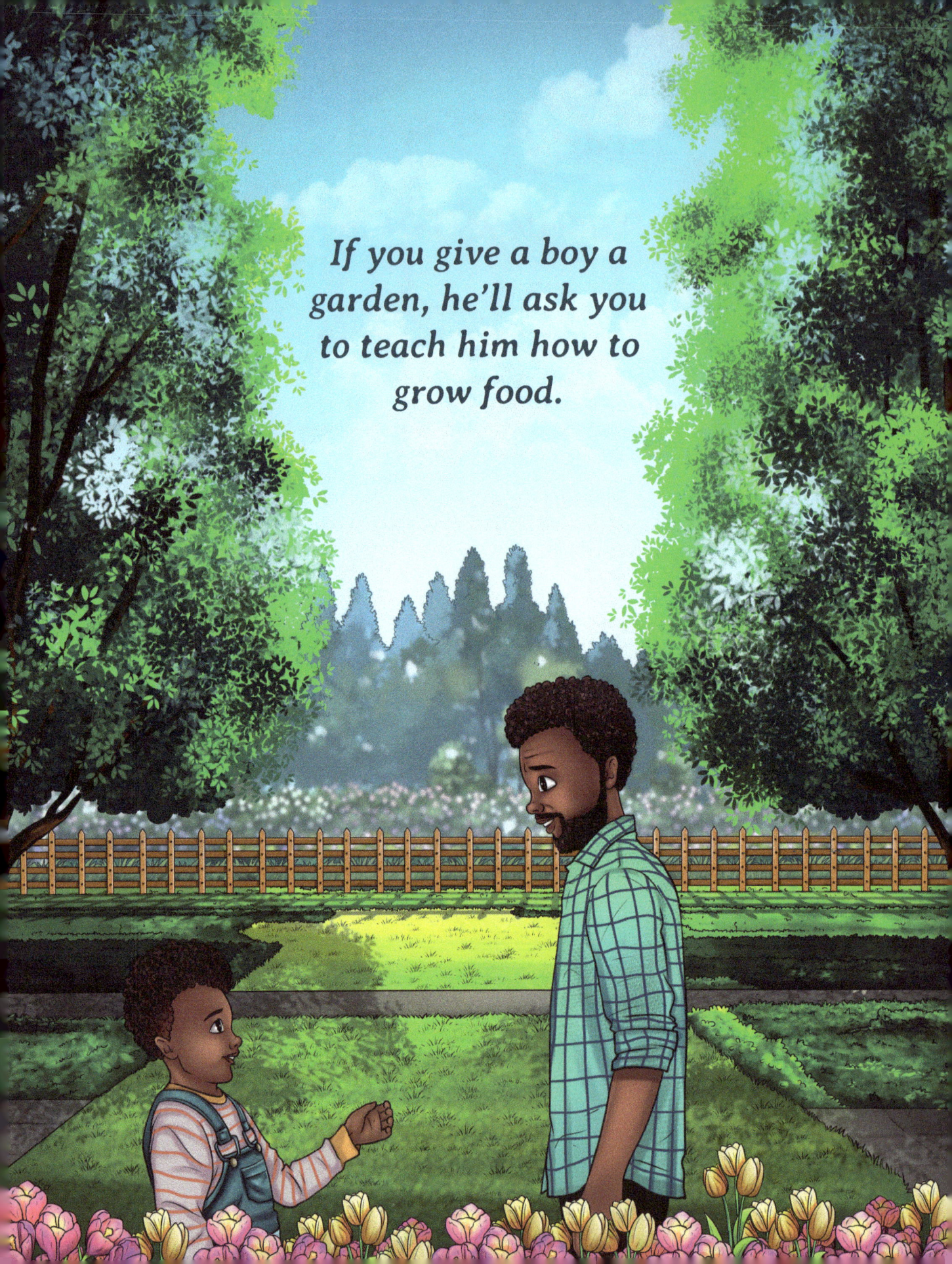

He'll want you to start at the beginning. From seed to supper, he wants to learn all the steps.

He will ask to go to the store to ensure he has all the proper tools and supplies.

Hardware Shop

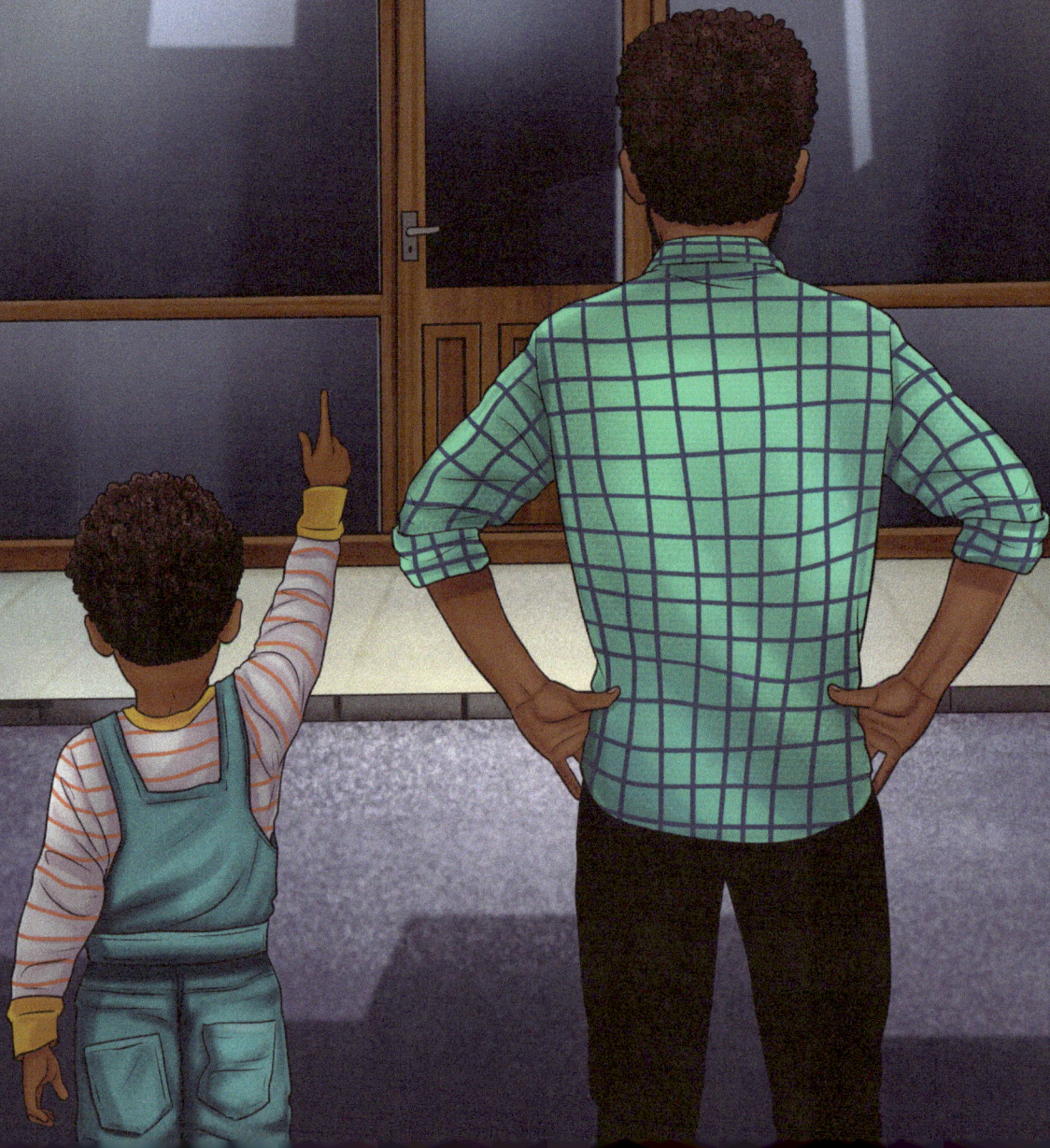

*When he has all the supplies, he will ask you how to plant the seeds for a successful harvest.*

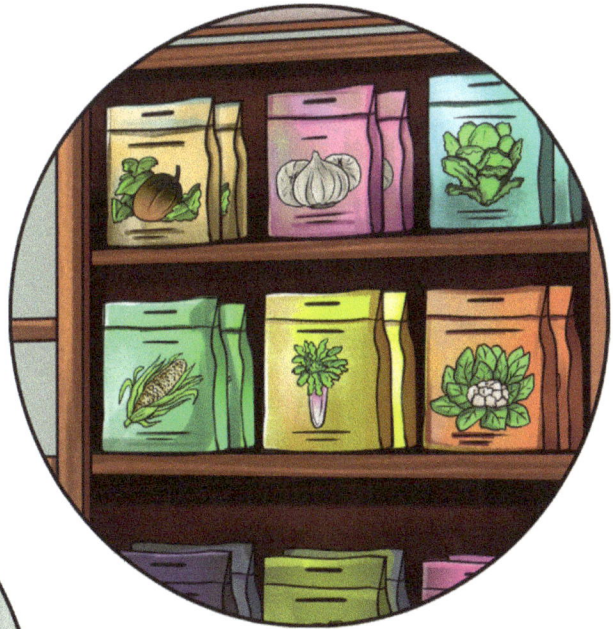

**Seeds**

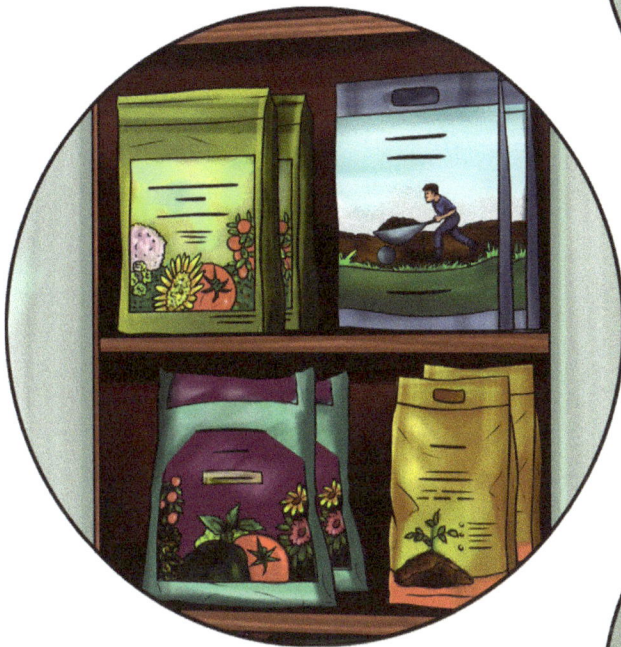

**Soil**

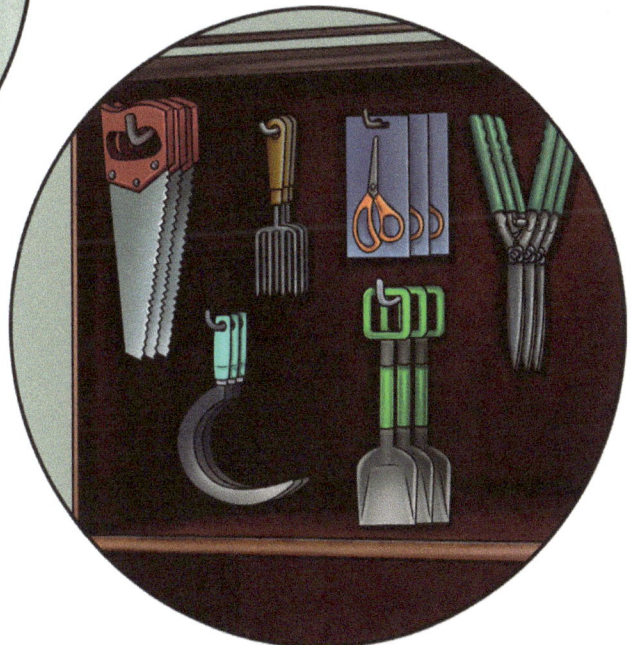

**Tools**

He'll want to learn about all the different techniques used to plant the crops.

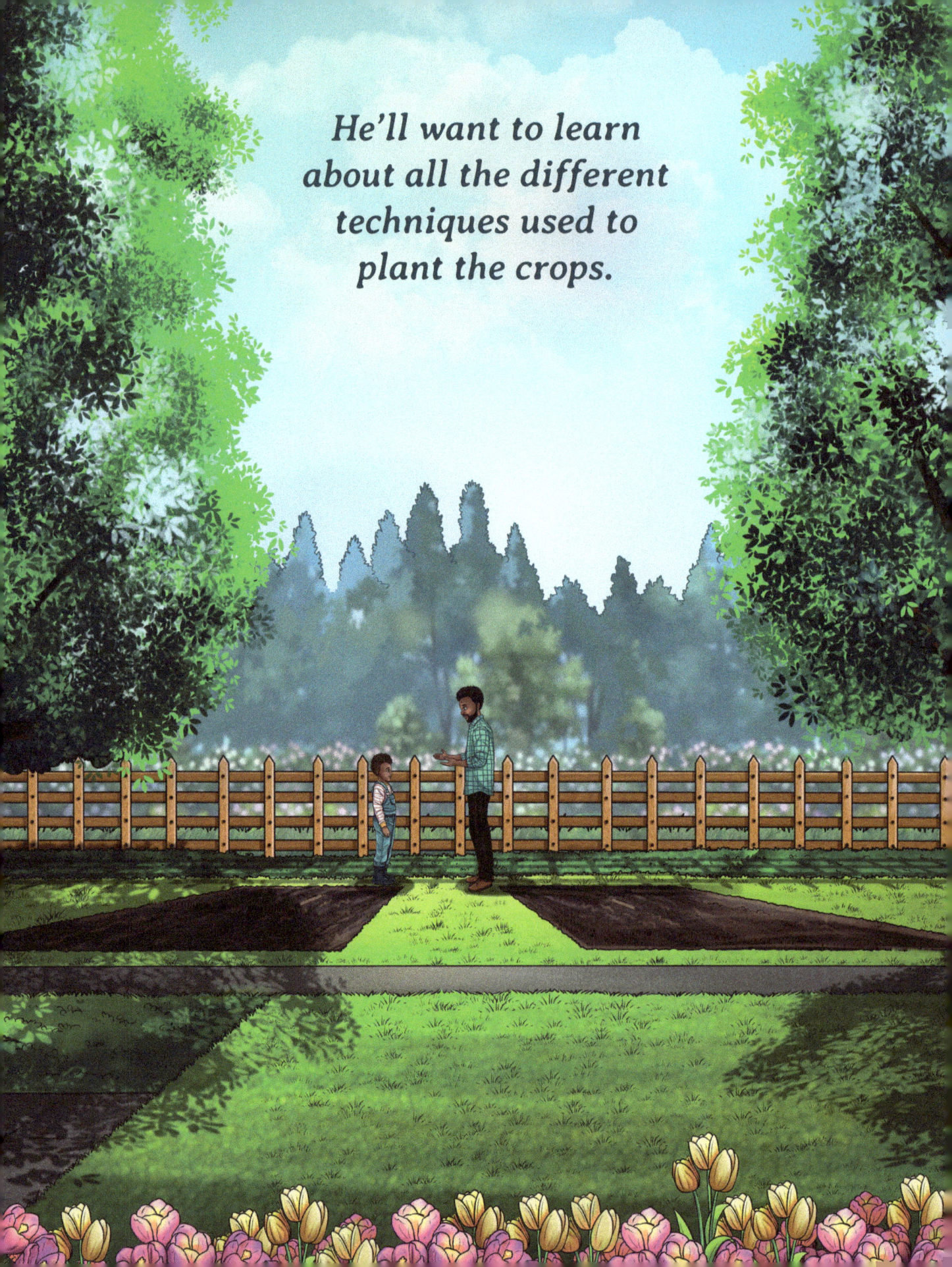

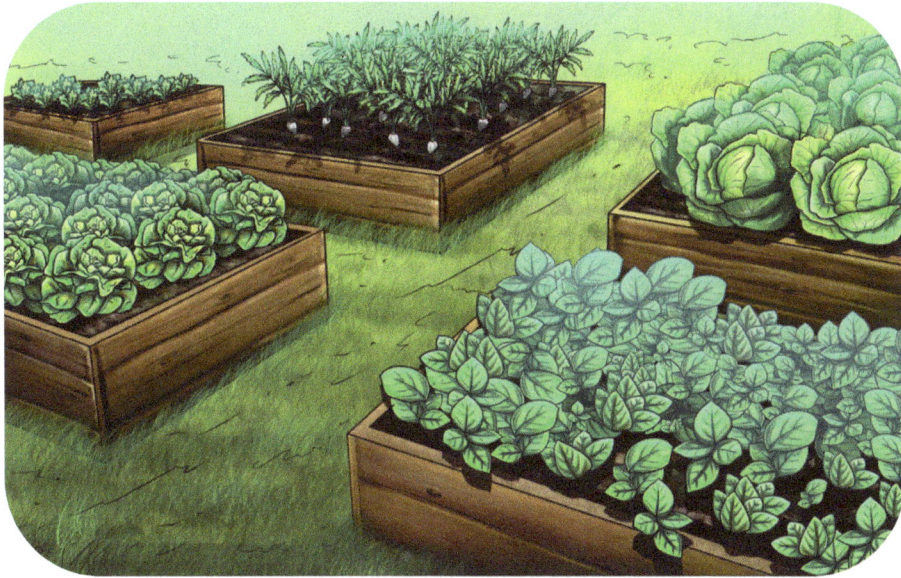

**Raised bed gardening**

**Vertical gardening**

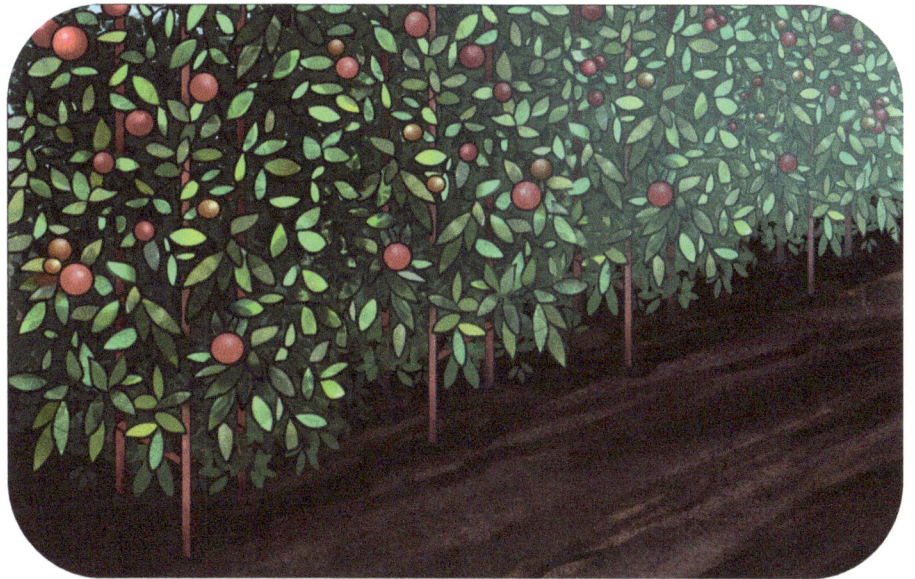

**Traditional in-ground gardening**

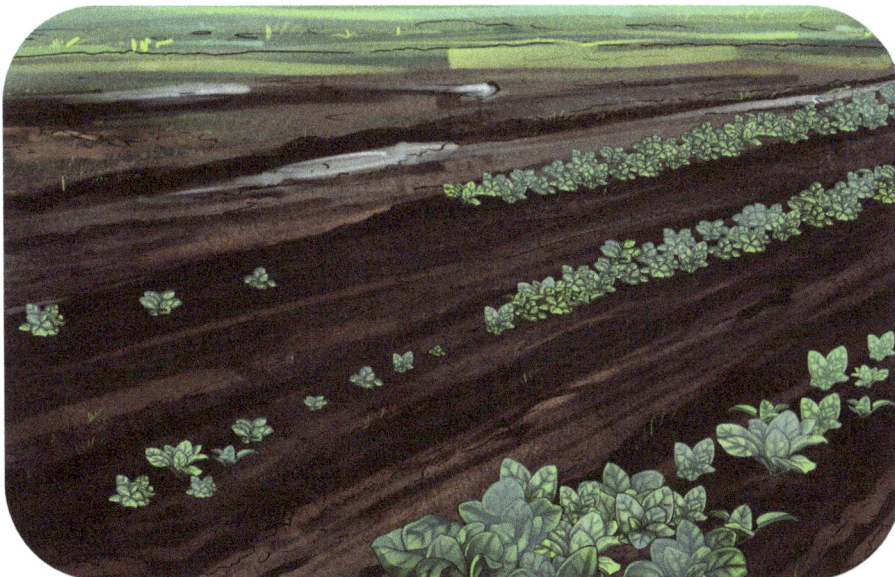

He'll probably ask which plants
to plant together and how far
apart each seed should be.

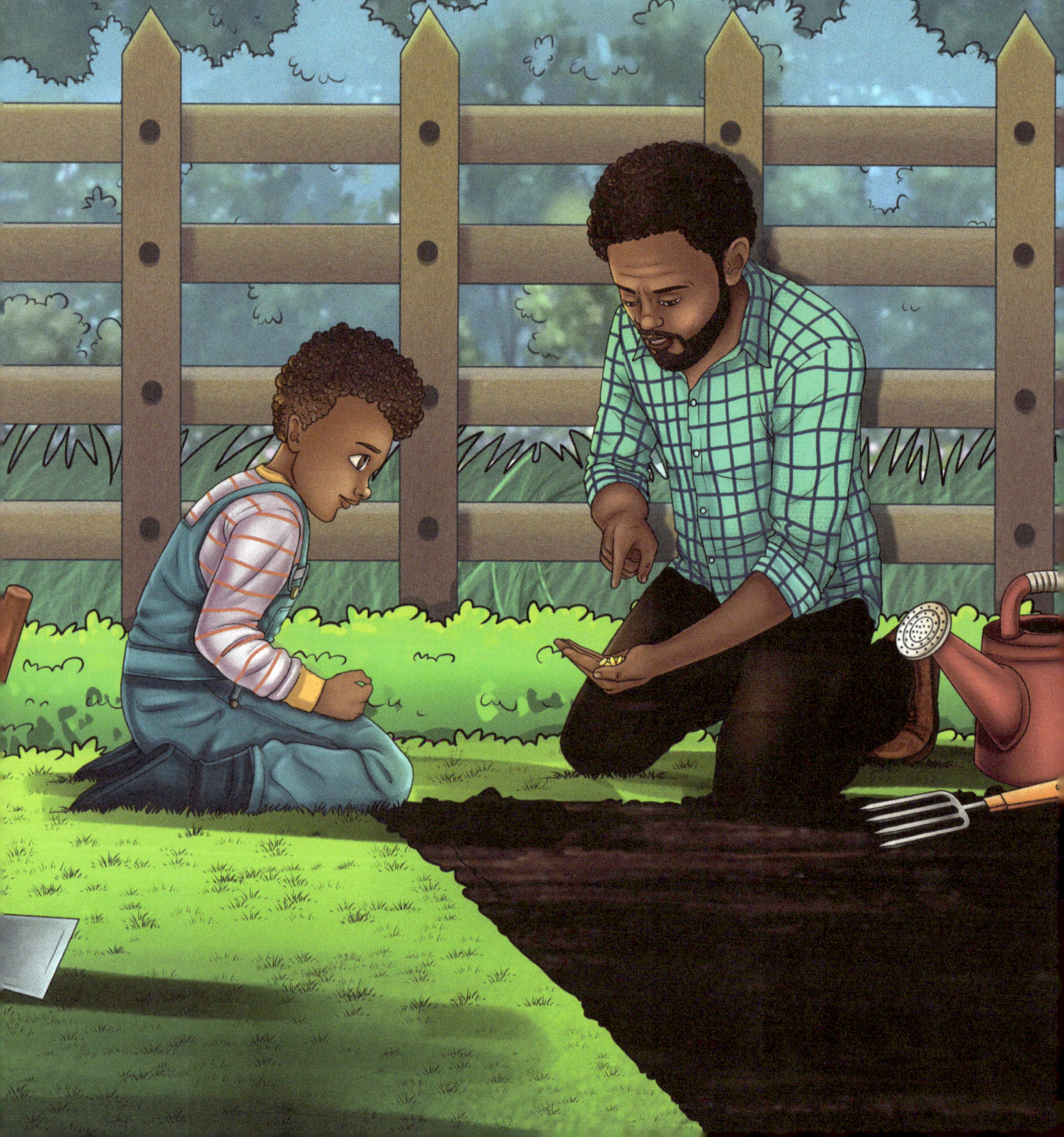

# Vegetable Spacing Guide

| | |
|---|---|
| **2-3" apart** | Bush peas, carrots, parsnips, peas, pole beans, radishes |
| **4-6" apart** | Beets, corn, garlic, kohlrabi, leeks, lettuce, spinach, onions |
| **6-10" apart** | Celery, peanuts, kale, swiss chard, mustard greens |
| **12-18" apart** | Cauliflower, cucumber, peppers, potatoes, sweet potatoes, zucchini |
| **18-24" apart** | Broccoli, cabbage, eggplant, fennel, tomatoes |
| **24" or more** | Melons, pumpkins, rhubarb, winter squash |

# Vegetable Opponents

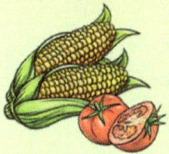

Corn & tomatoes

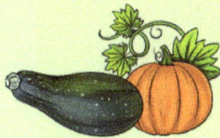

Summer squash & pumpkins

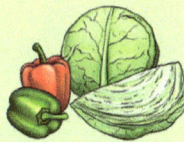

Peppers & cabbage

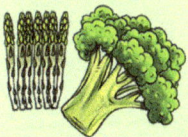

Asparagus & broccoli

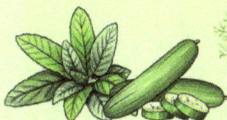

Sage & cucumber

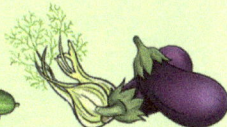

Fennel & eggplant

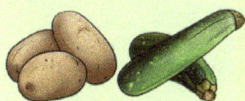

Potatoes & zucchini

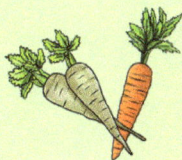

Carrots & parsnips

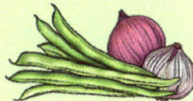

Beans & onions

# Companion Planting Guide

**Radishes**
Cucumbers, carrots, onions, beets, cabbage, kale, lettuce, spinach, squash

**Corn**
Green beans, cucumbers, peas, pumpkins, melons, squash

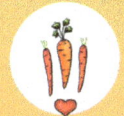

**Carrots**
Tomatoes, leeks, rosemary, sage, chives

**Tomatoes**
Basil, carrots, asparagus, celery, onions, lettuce, parsley, spinach

**Cucumbers**
Beans, celery, corn, lettuce, dill, peas, radishes

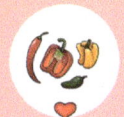

**Peppers**
Onions, tomatoes, spinach, basil

**Lettuce**
Chives, corn, garlic, peas, beans, beets, broccoli, carrots

**Onions**
Carrots, cabbage, lettuce, tomatoes, parsnips

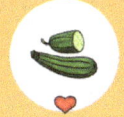

**Squash**
Corn, beans, peas, radishes, dill

Once he has planted the seeds,
he'll ask how to label the crops
to identify all the garden rows.

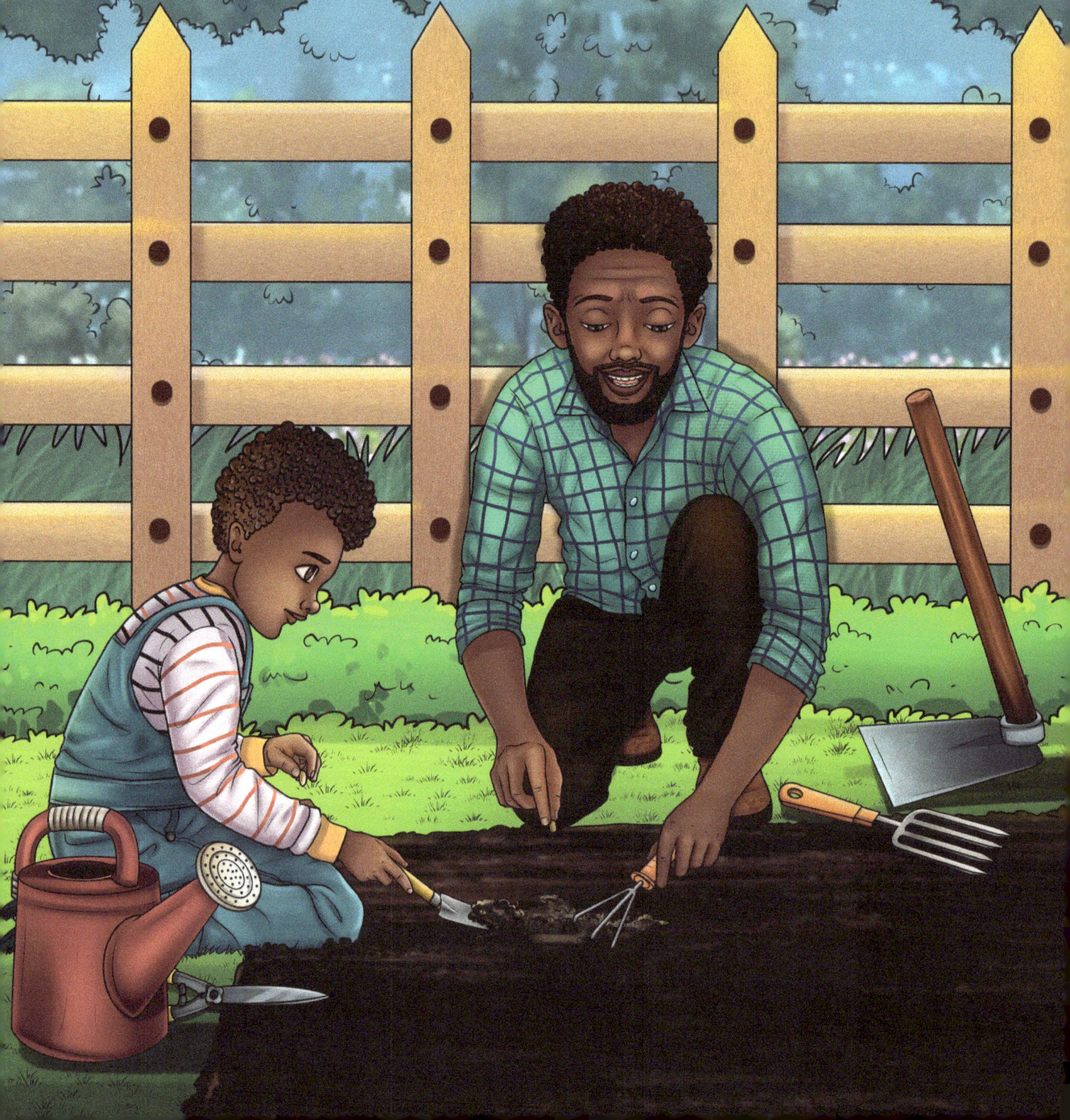

After labeling the garden rows, he will need to learn how to maintain his food forest.

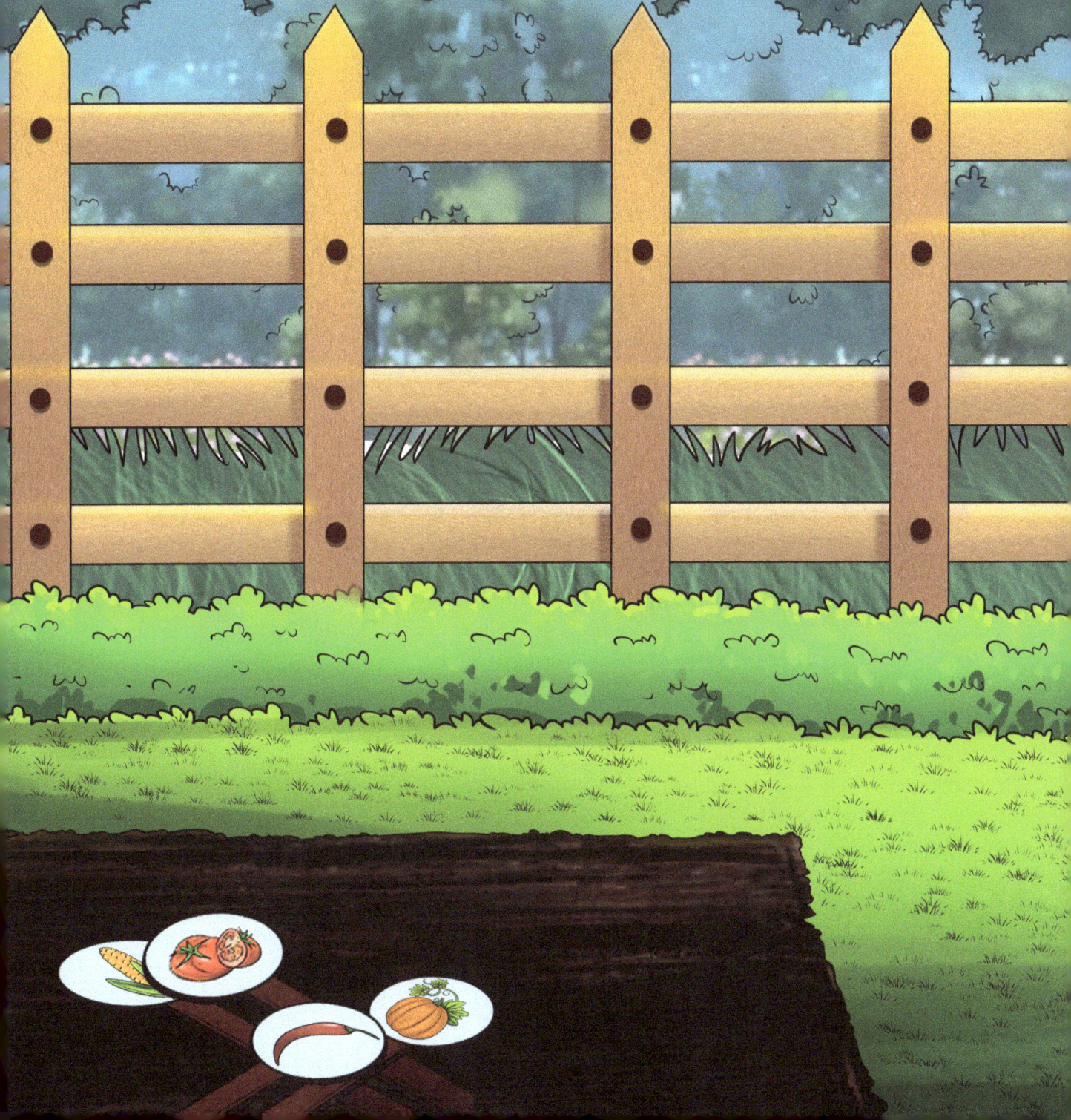

He will ask you to teach him the watering schedule to ensure the crops have plenty of water to grow.

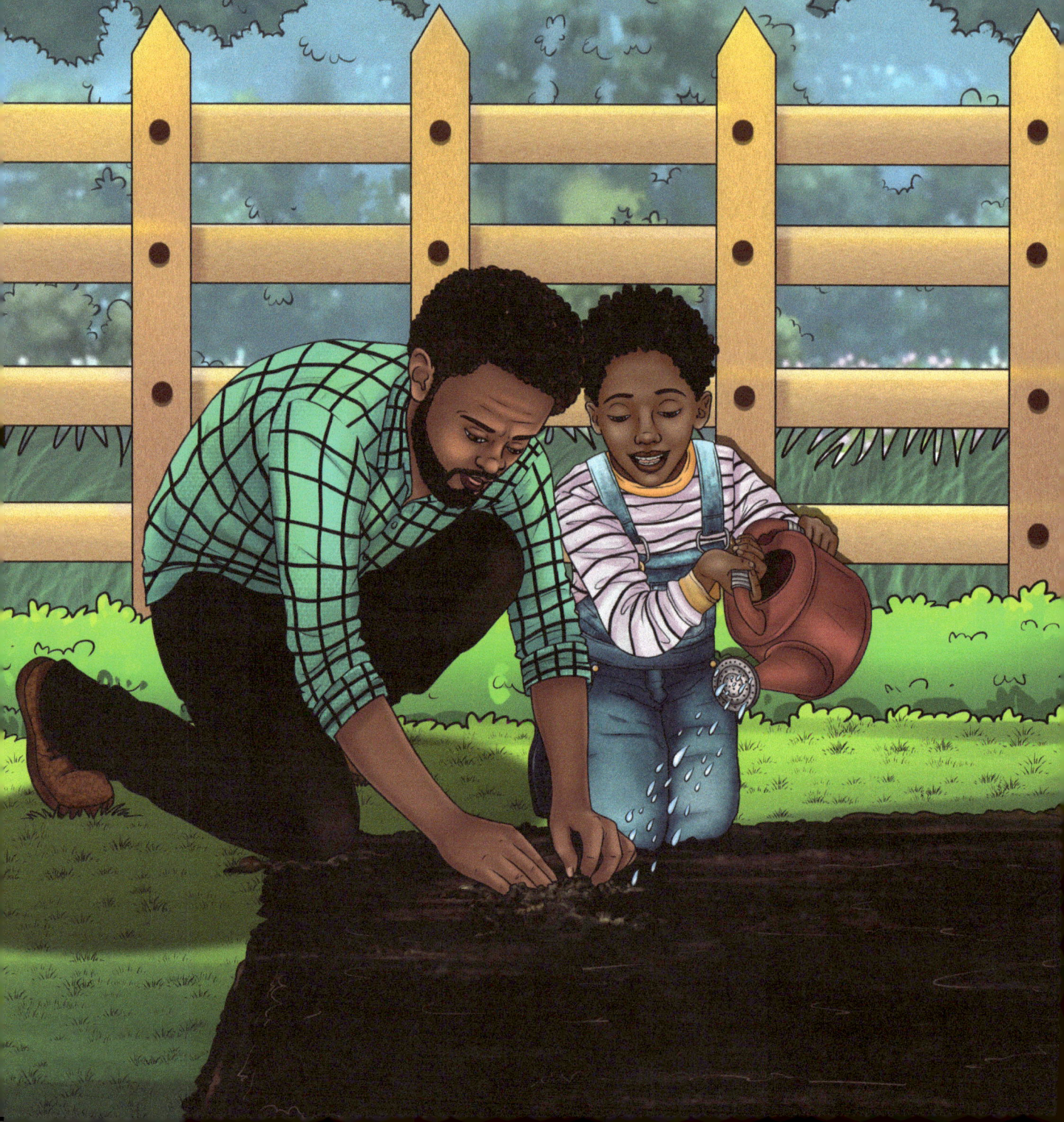

# Garden Watering Schedule

| Twice a week | Once a week | 10 Days to 2 weeks |
|---|---|---|
| Lettuce | Beans | Tomatoes |
| Celery | Corn | Watermelons |
| Spinach | Peppers | Cantaloupes |
| Swiss Chard | Eggplant | Butternut Squash |
| Radishes | Zucchini | Hubbard Squash |
| Beets | Summer Squash | Banana Squash |
| Carrots | Cucumbers | Peaches |
| Turnips | Yams | Nectarines |
| Potatoes | Peanuts | Pears |
| Broccoli | Rhubarb | Apples |
| Cauliflower | Onions | Plums |
| Strawberries | Pumpkins | Cherries |
| Raspberries | | Grapes |
| Blackberries | | Asparagus |
| Peas | | |

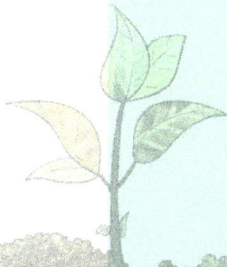
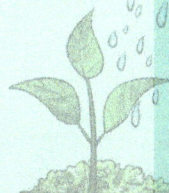
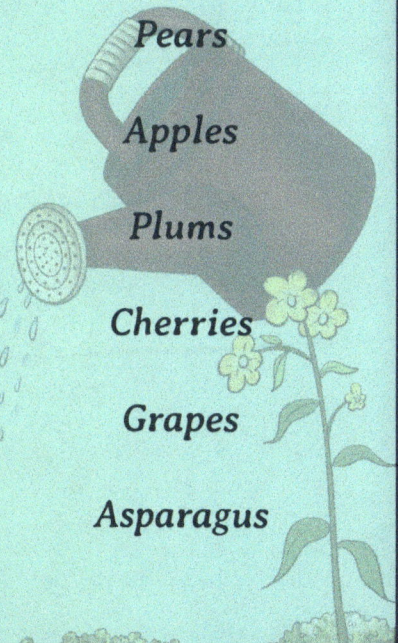

Then he will ask you to teach
him how to groom the garden.

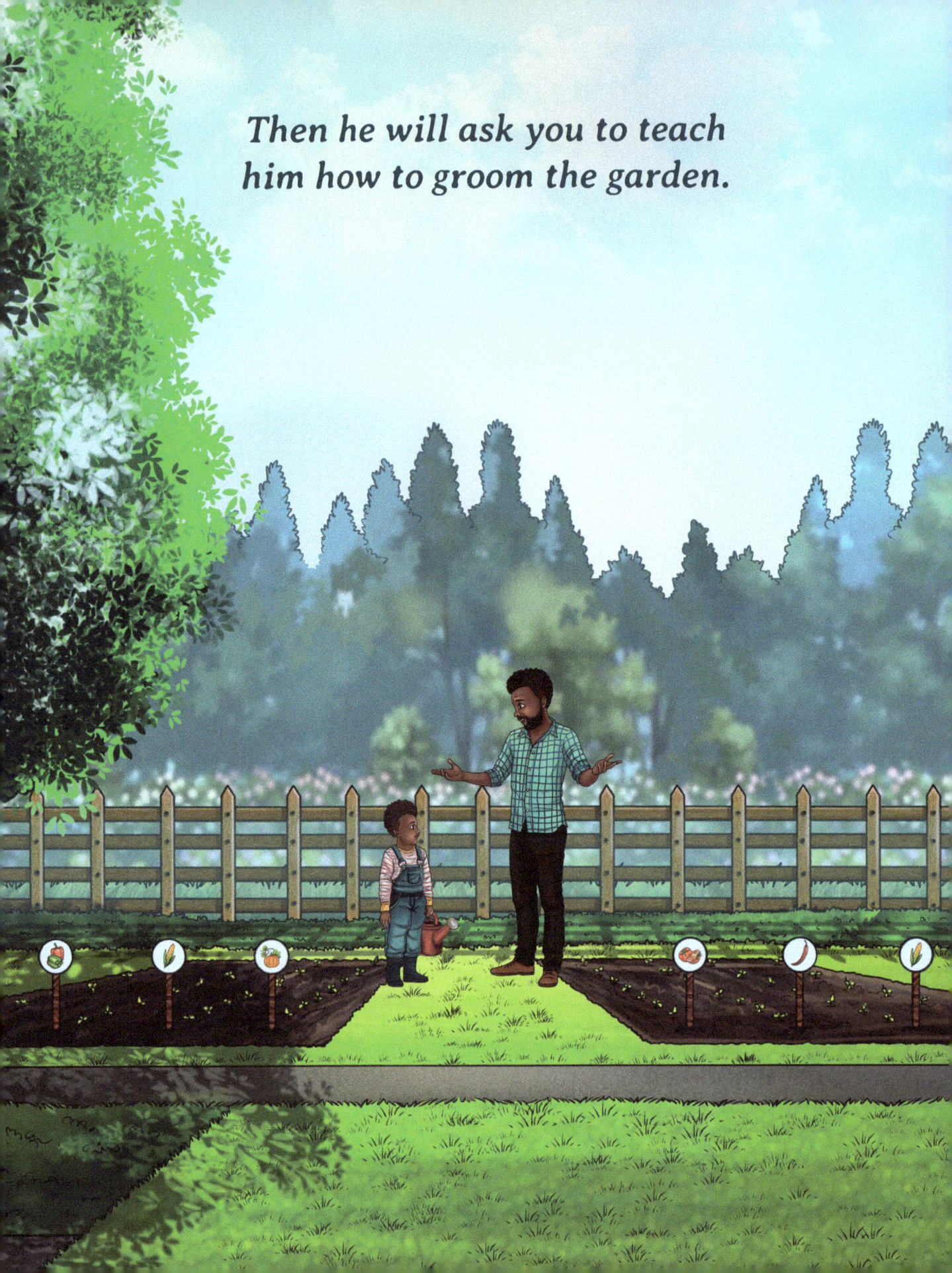

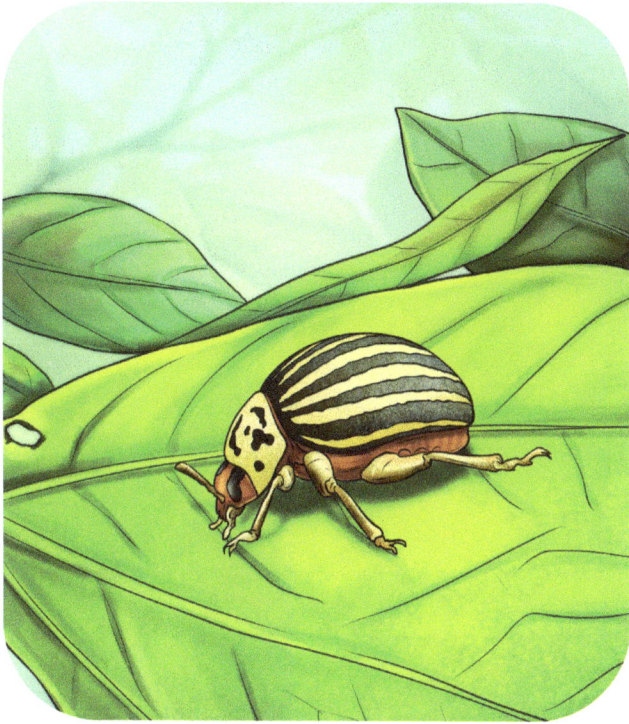

**Watch out for bugs**

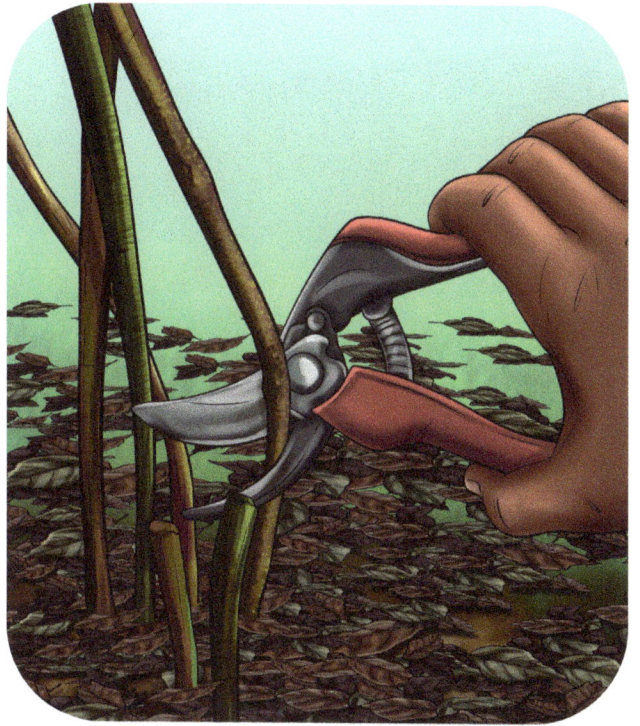

**Trim damaged leaves**

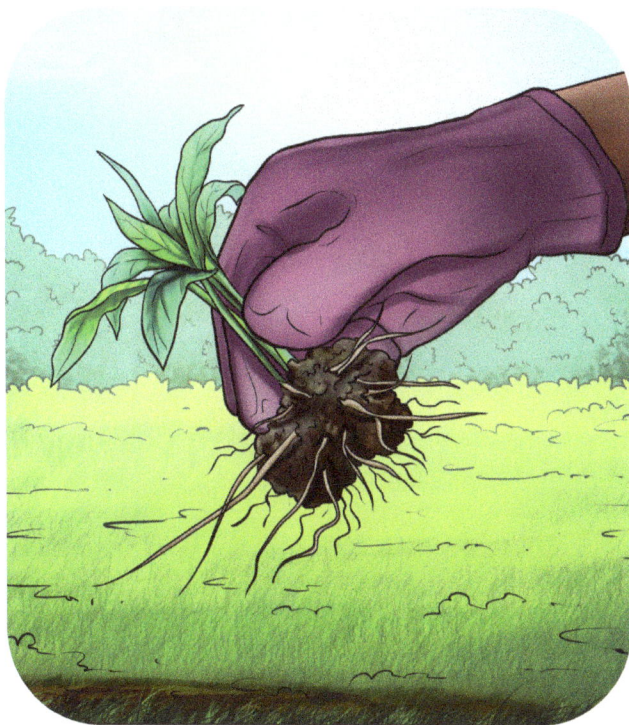

**Pull weeds**

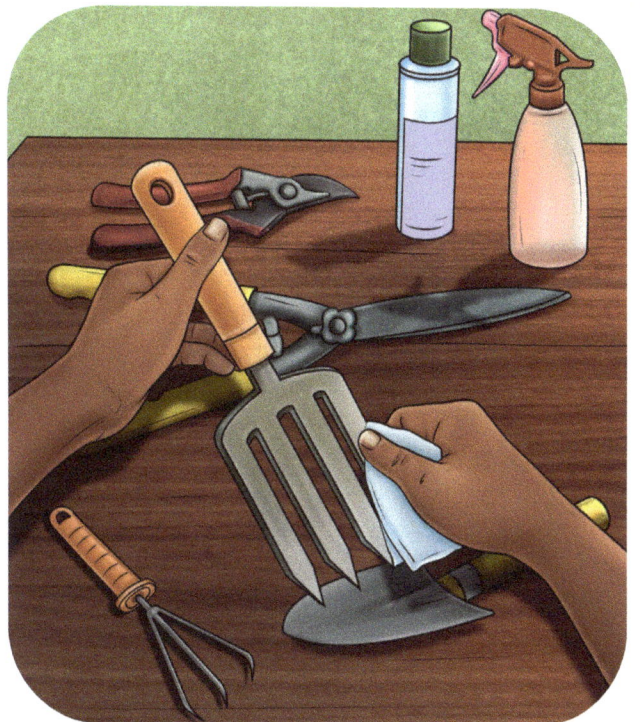

**Clean gardening tools**

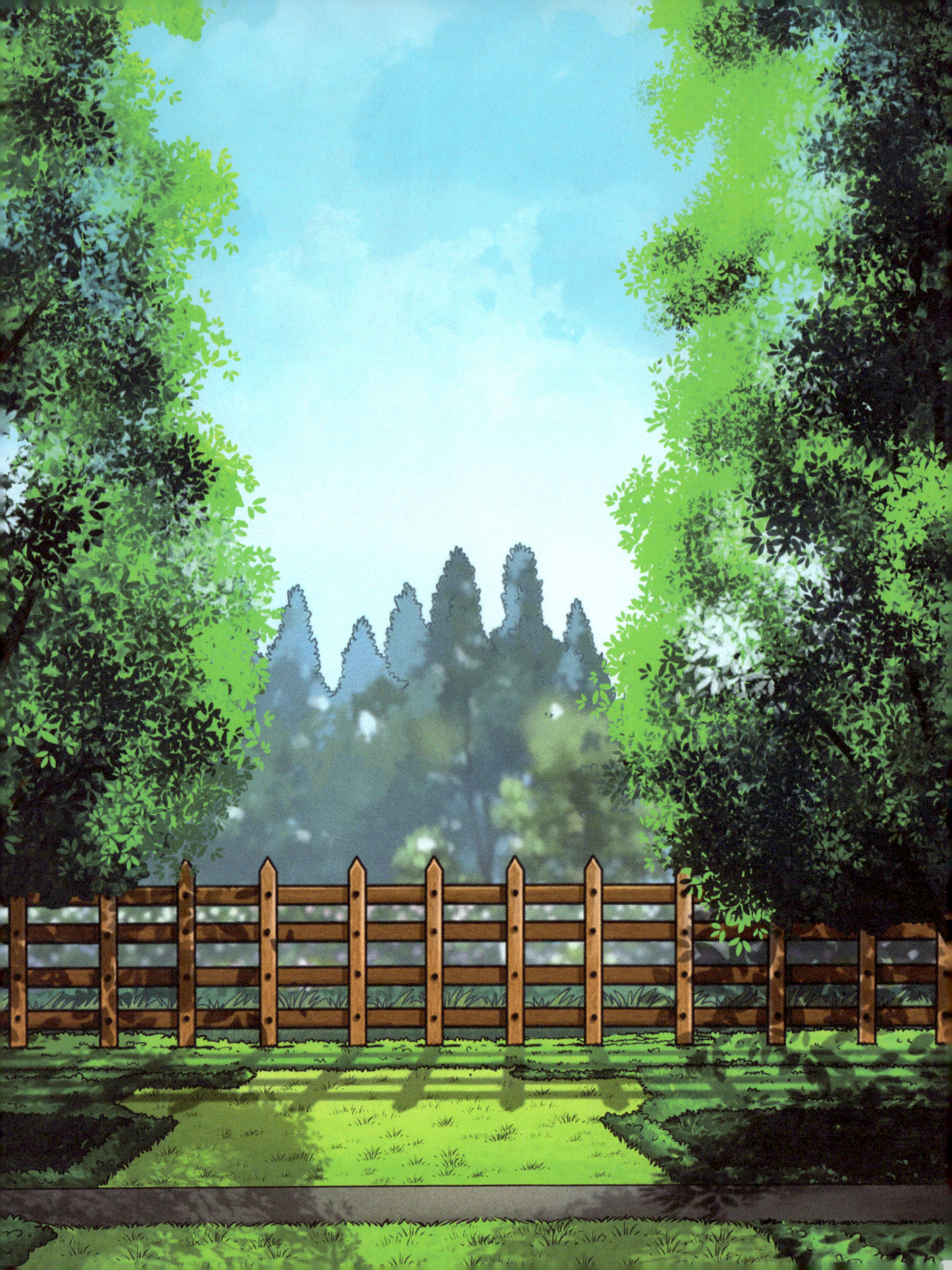

When he sees the garden growing
and food appearing, he will know
he is learning the best practices
for taking care of a garden.

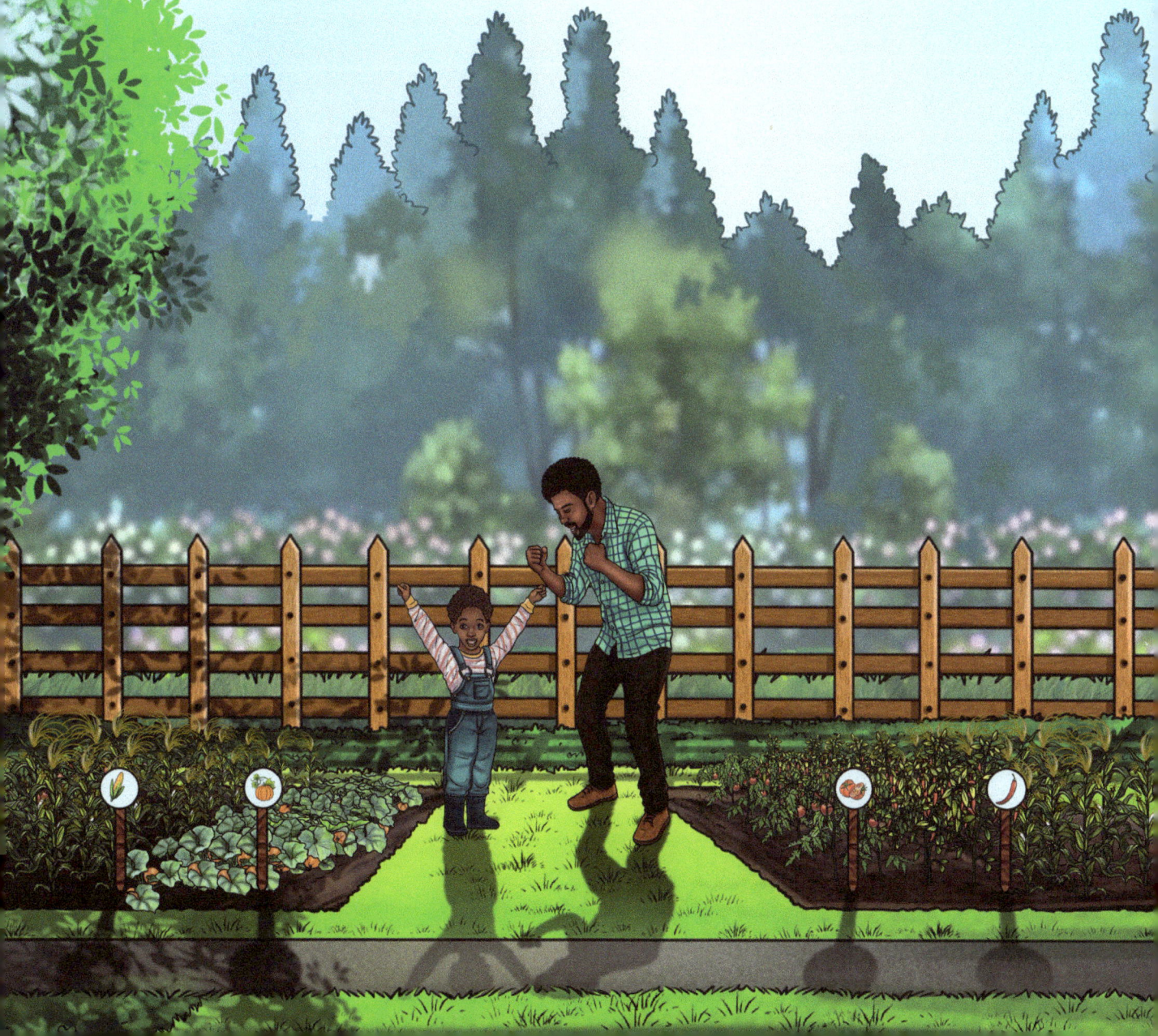

Once the crops have grown for a few months, he'll want to know the best time to harvest the crops.

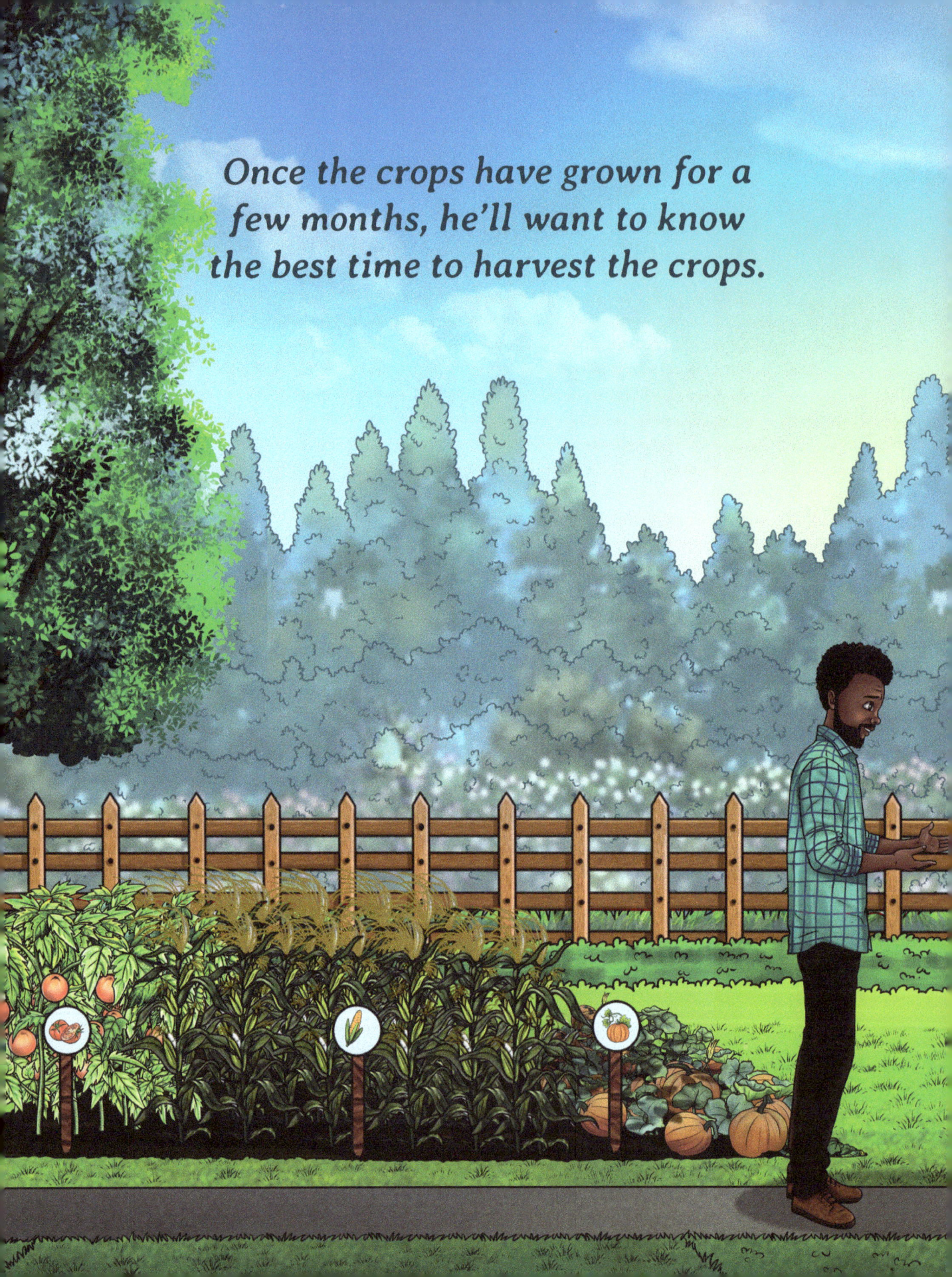

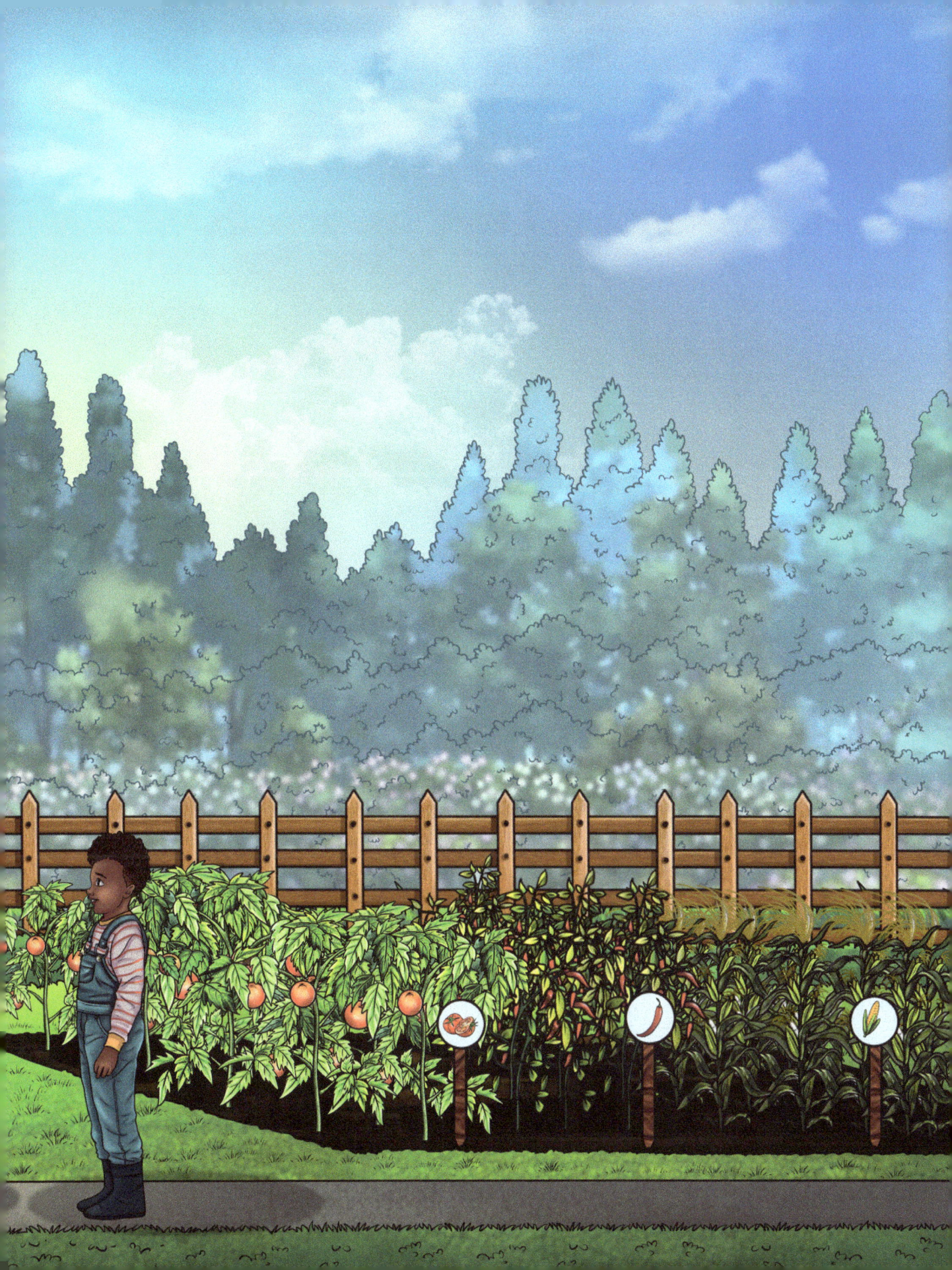

*He will ask for an explanation about all the best harvesting methods.*

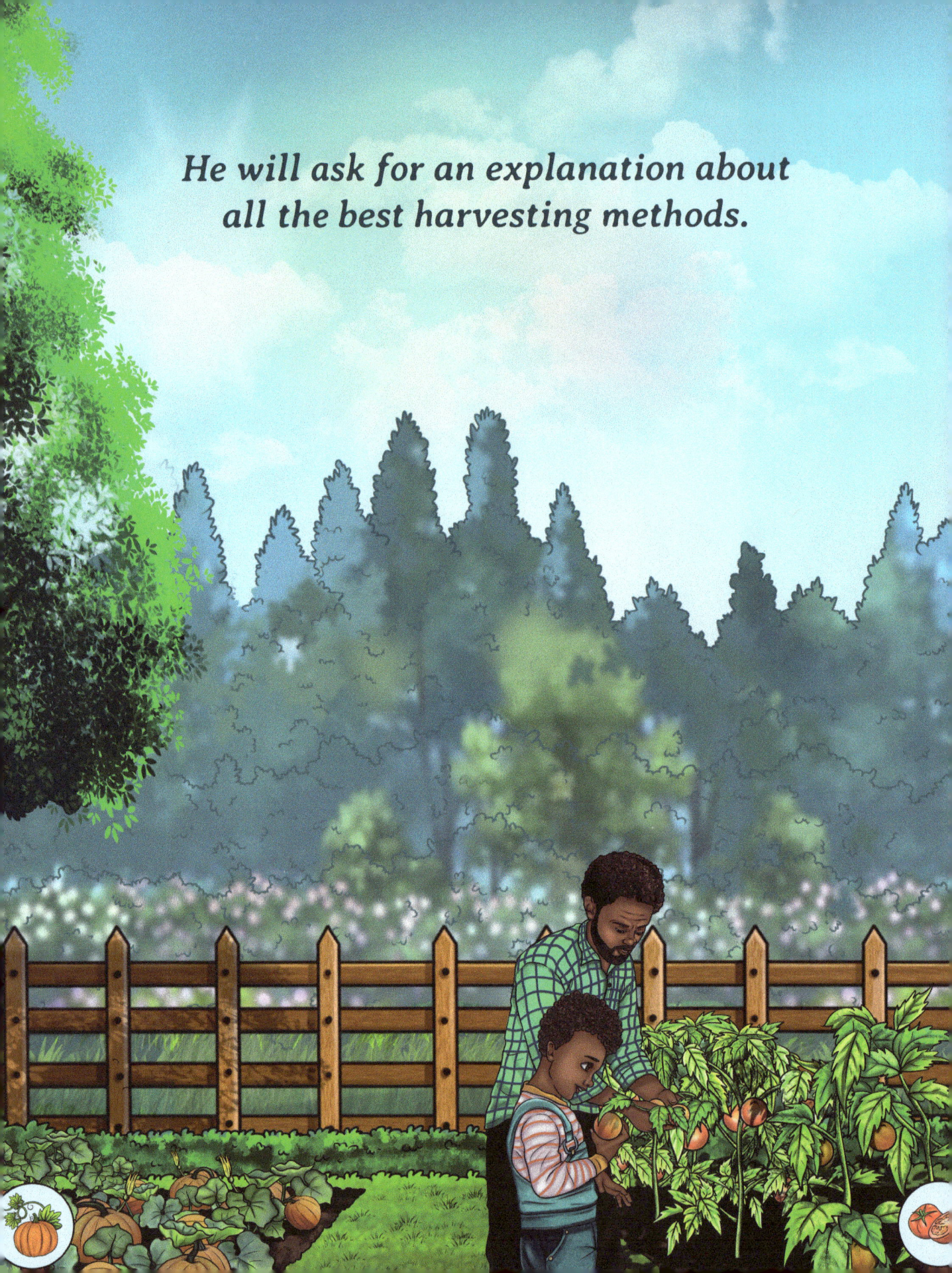

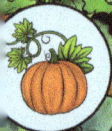

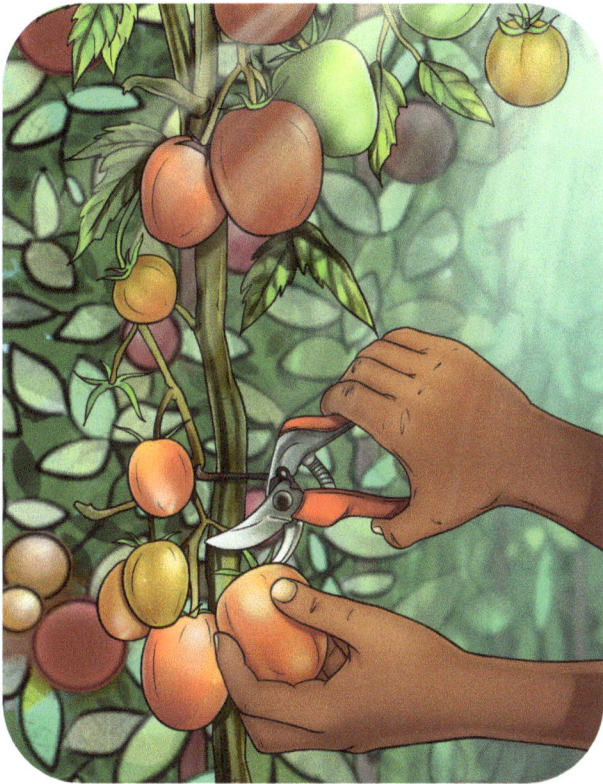

**Two hands when picking**

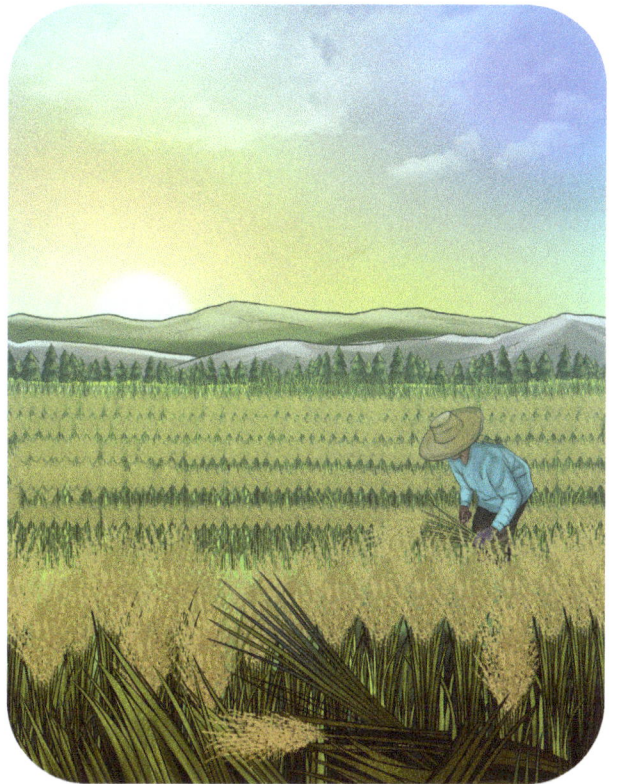

**Harvest in the morning**

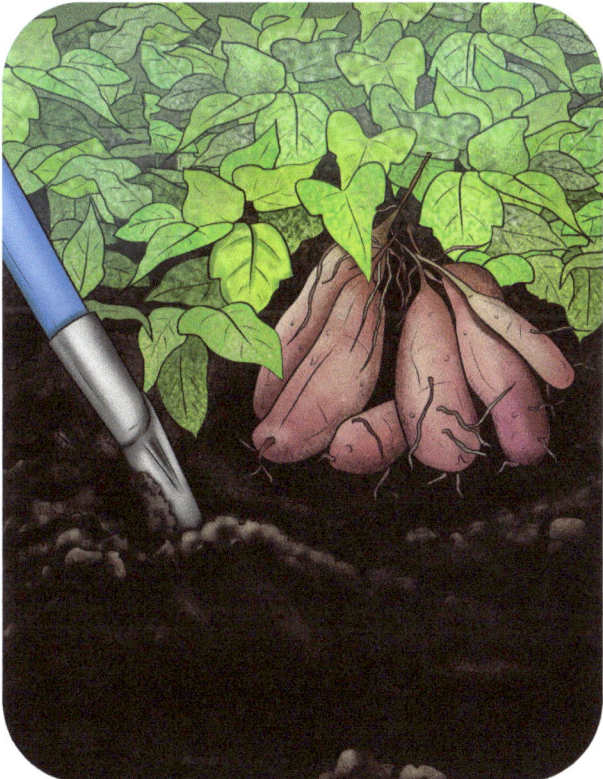

**Harvesting with tools**

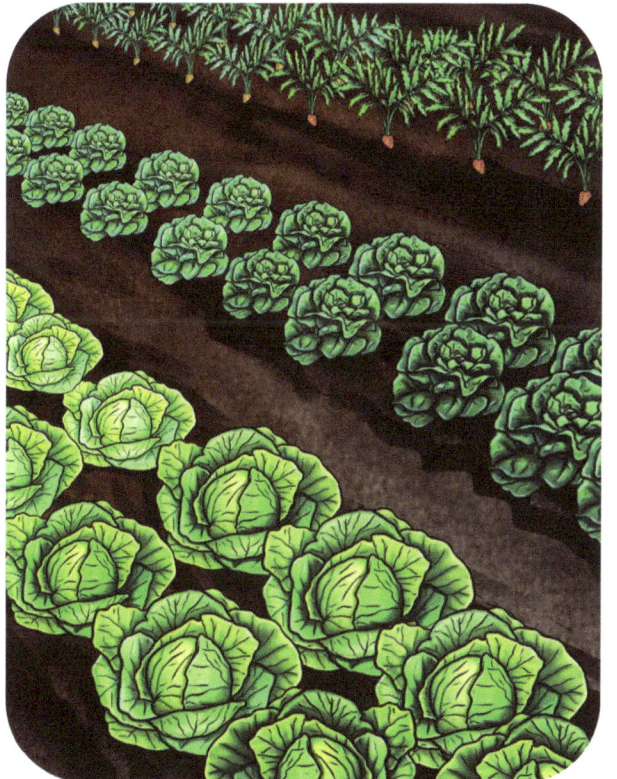

**Size matters**

Once the crops have been harvested, he will want to know how to store the food.

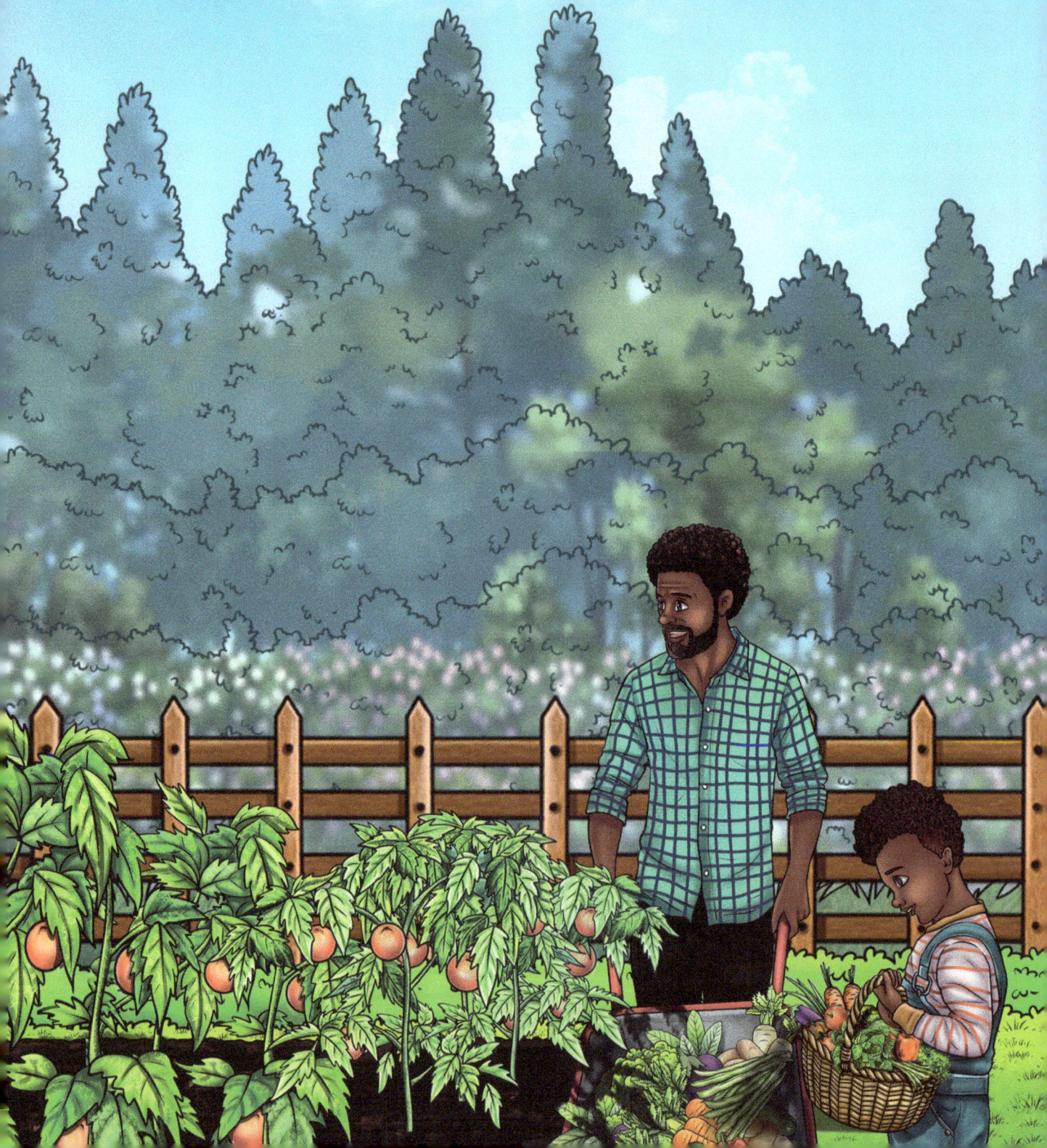

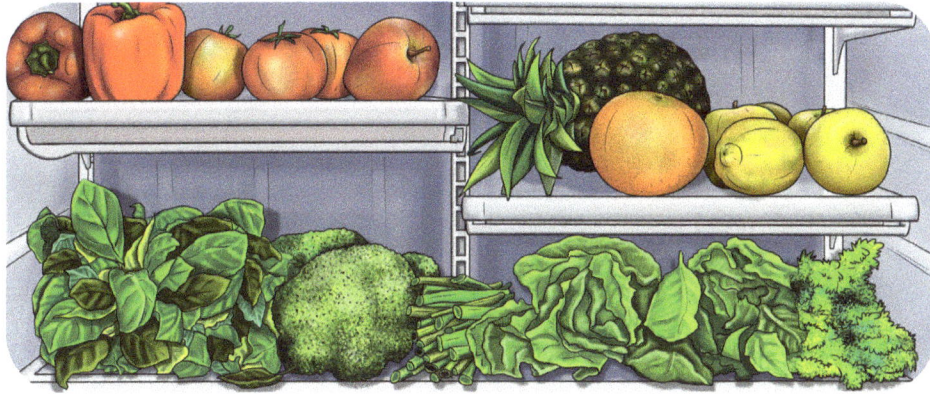

**Refrigerate or freeze your surplus**

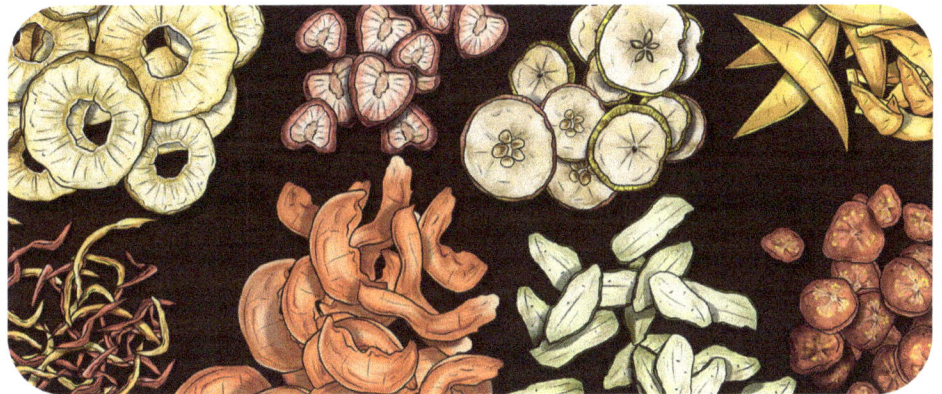

**Dehydrate**

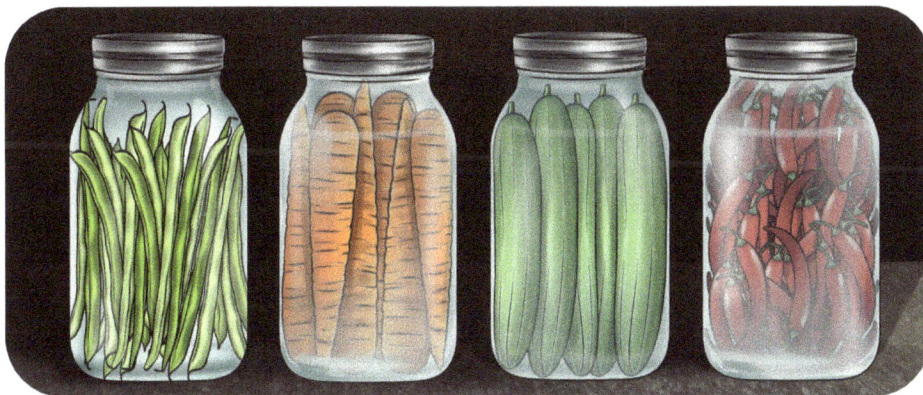

**Canning**

*Seeing that he has plenty of fruits and vegetables, he'll want to share with neighbors and give them tips on how to store the food.*

*After months of hard work, he'll want to enjoy the fruits of his labor.*

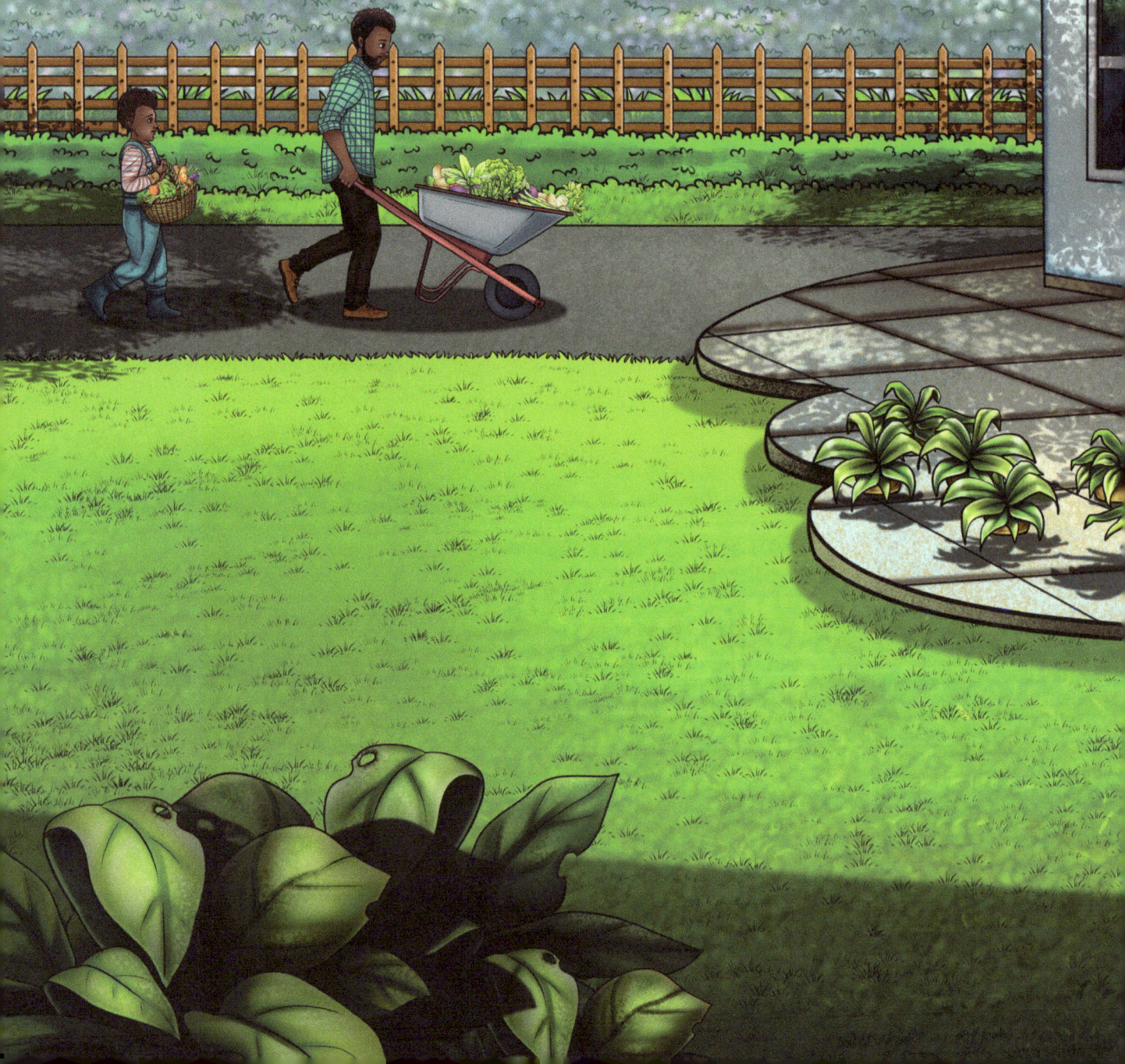

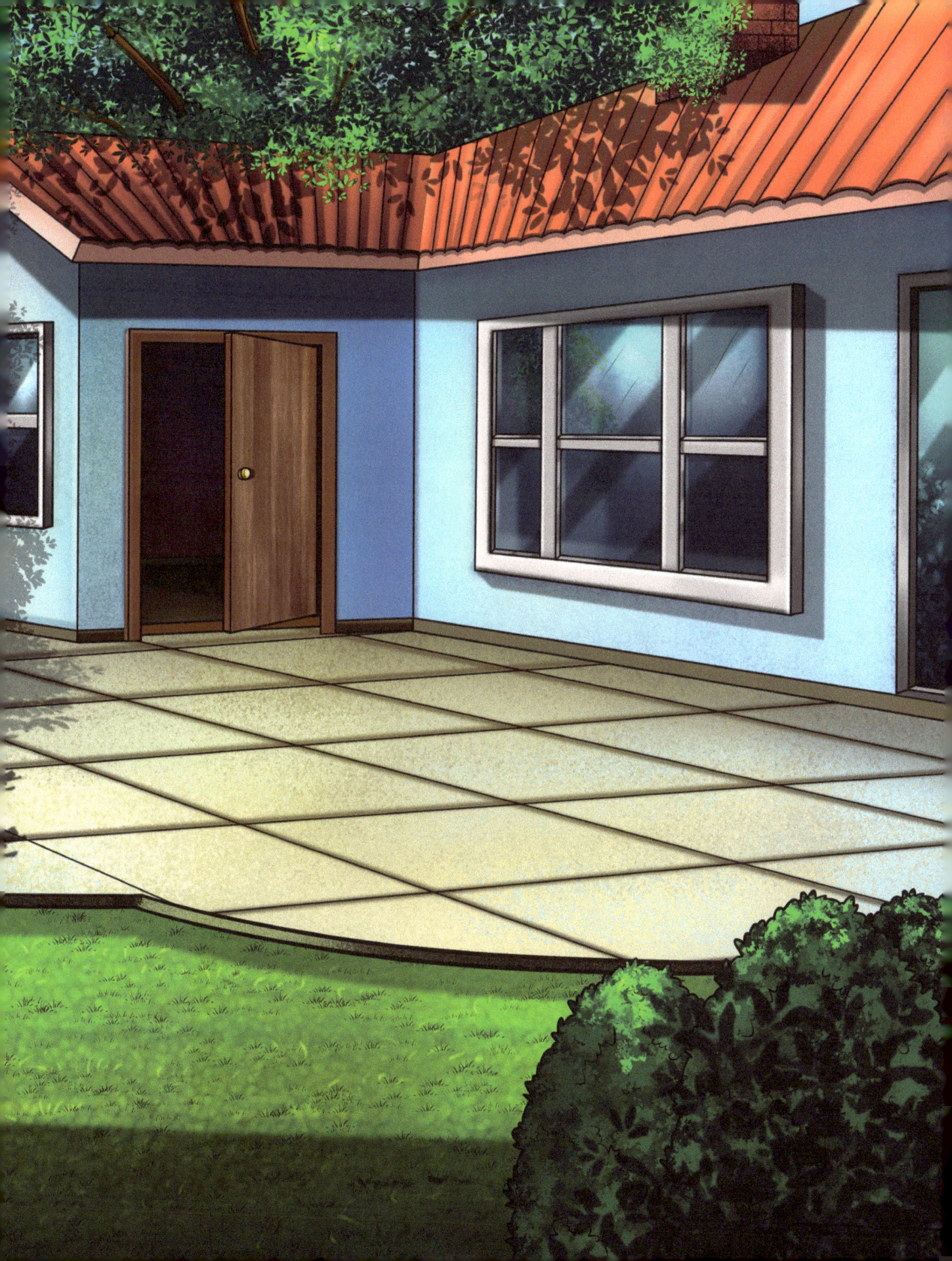

*He'll ask you to cook some of the food from the garden for supper.*

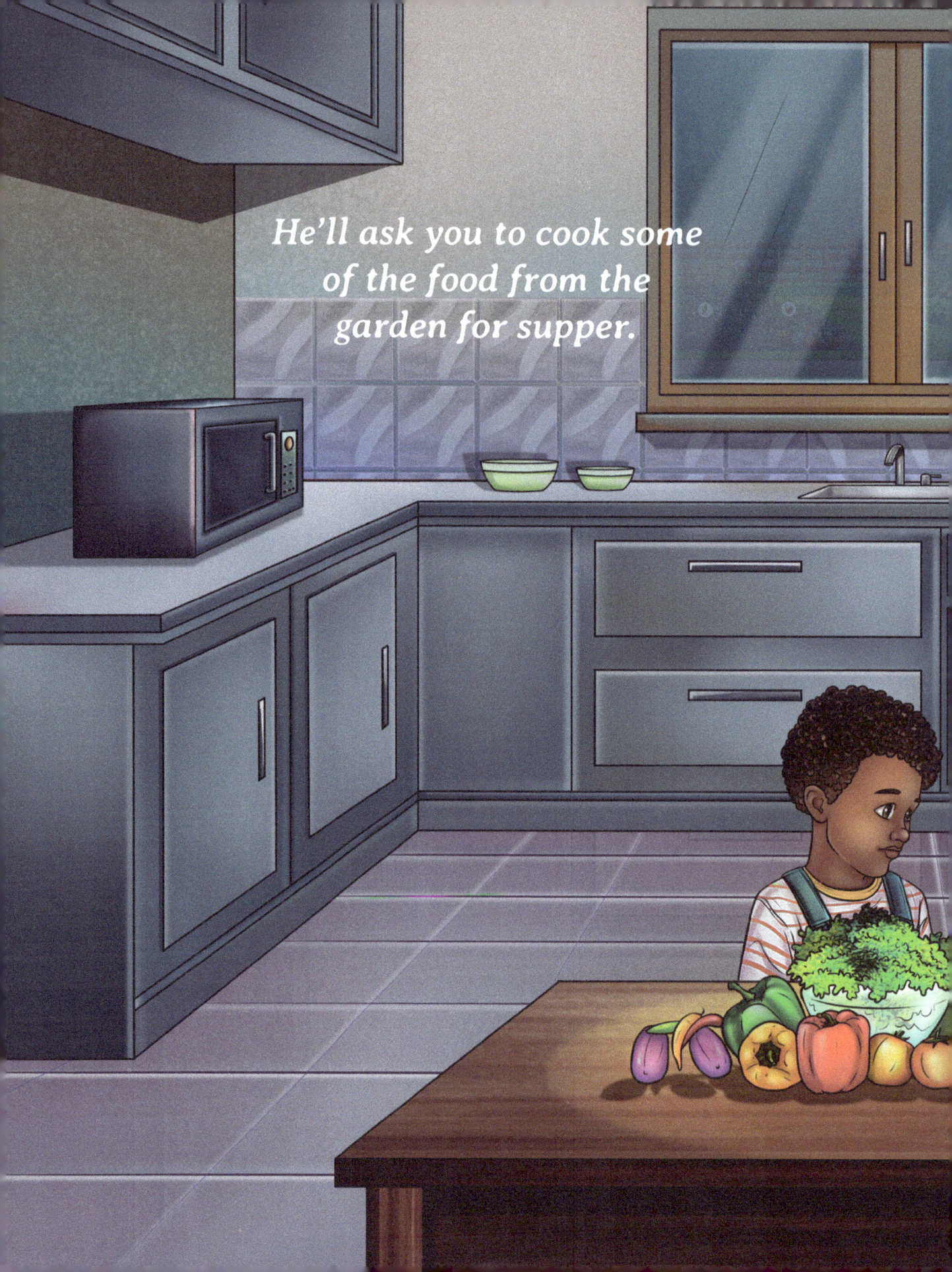

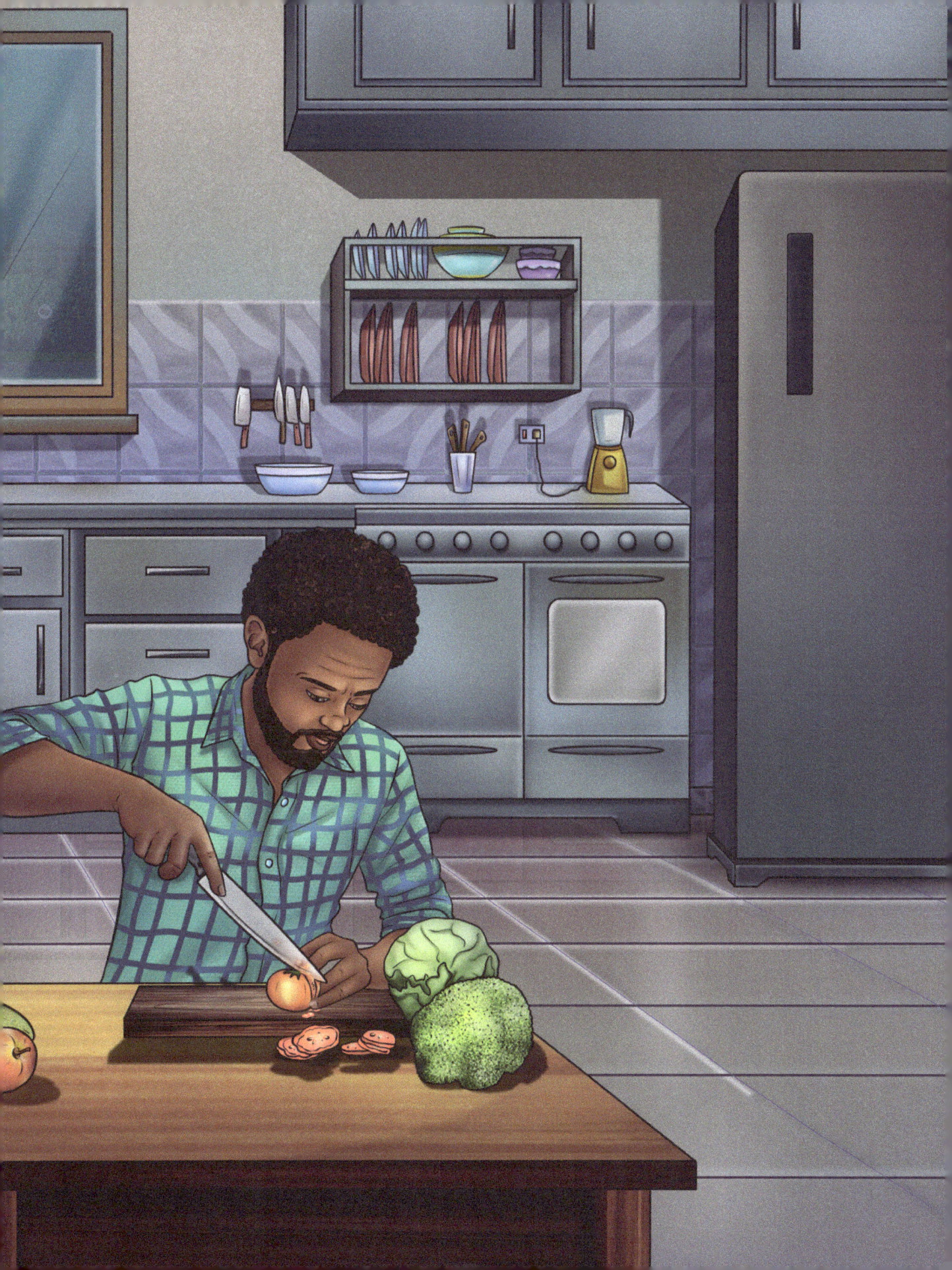

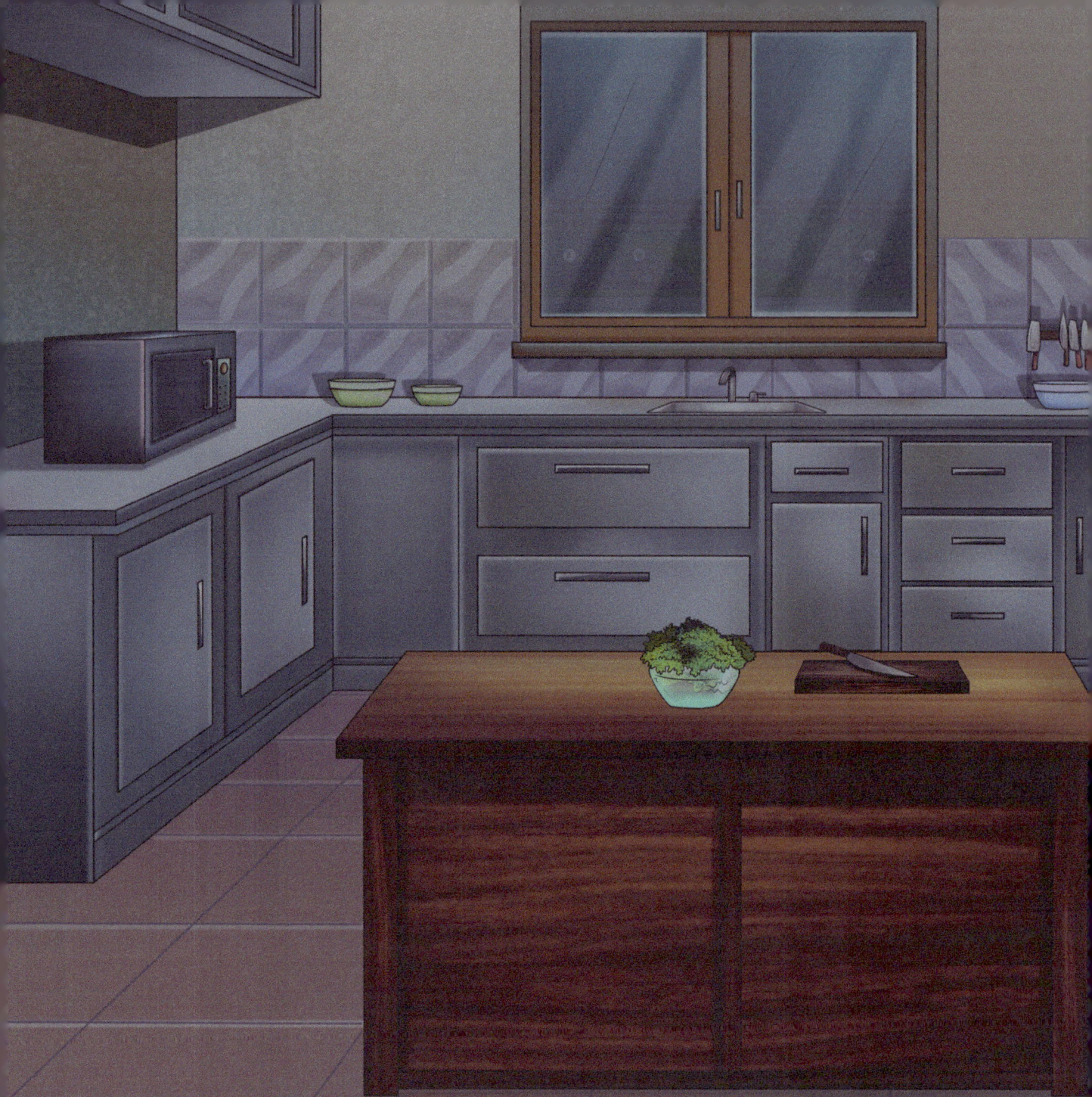

Then he will sit down with his family and enjoy the delicious food he grew.

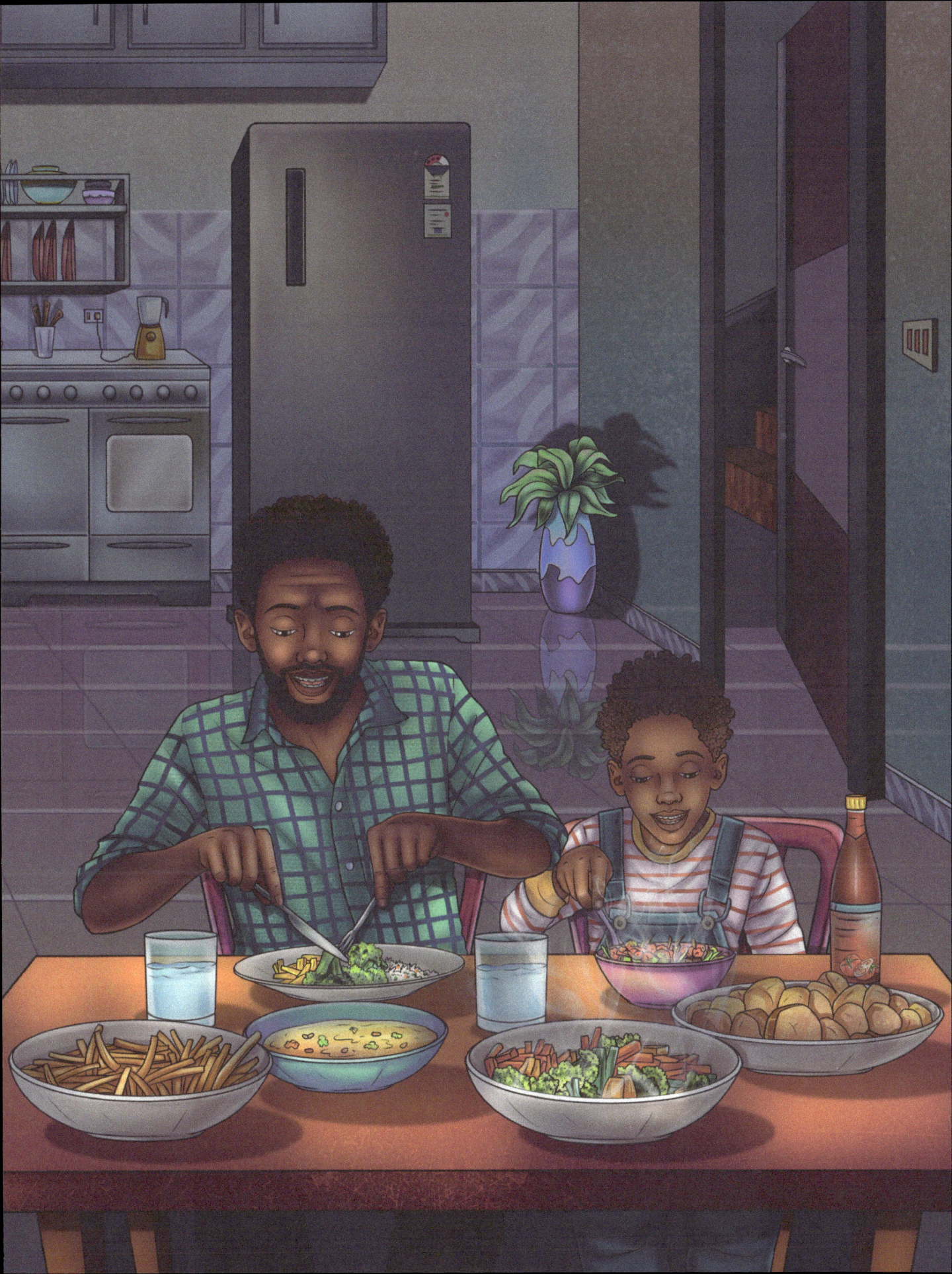

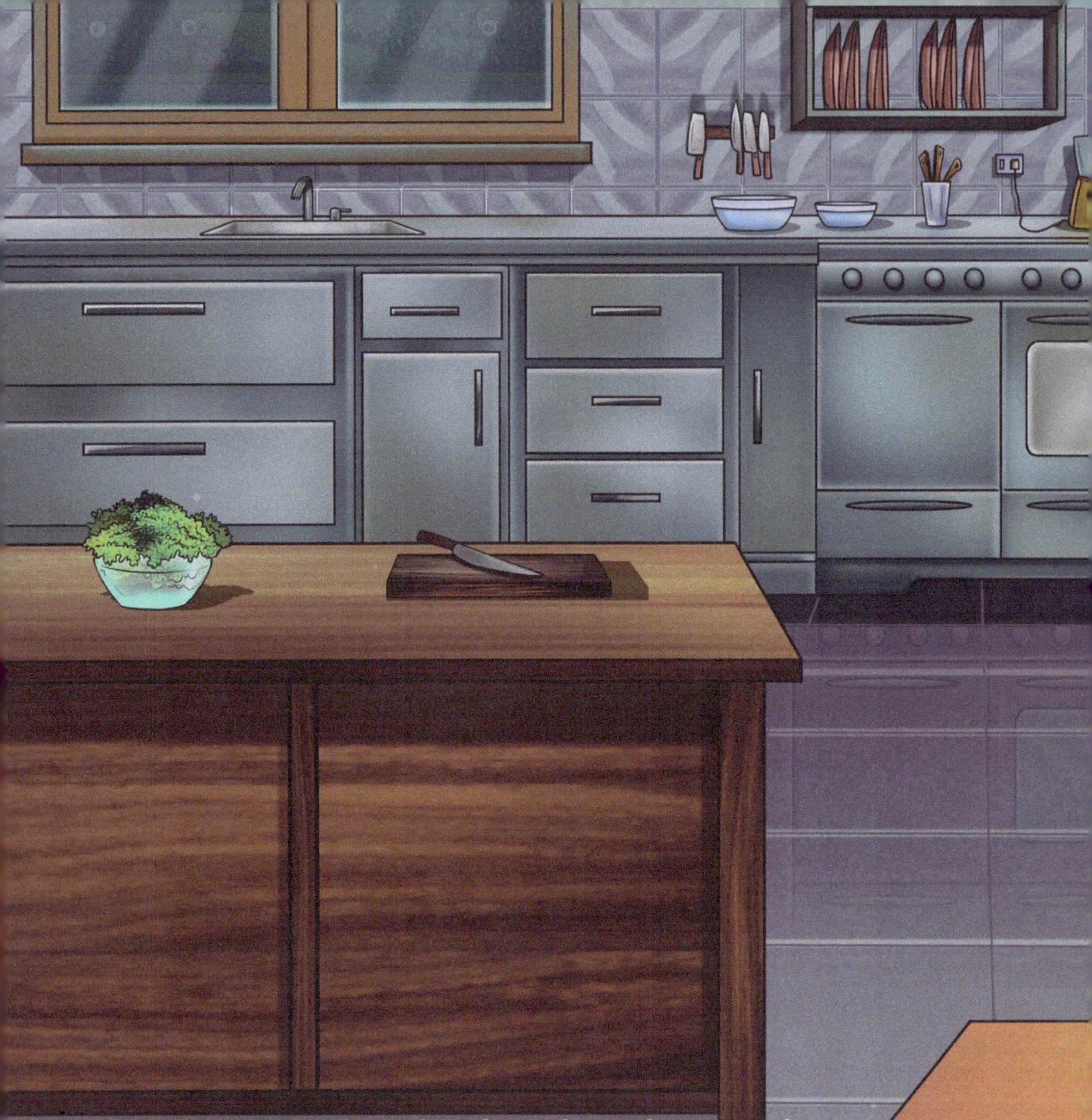

When he finishes dinner, he will thank you for helping him become a gardener.

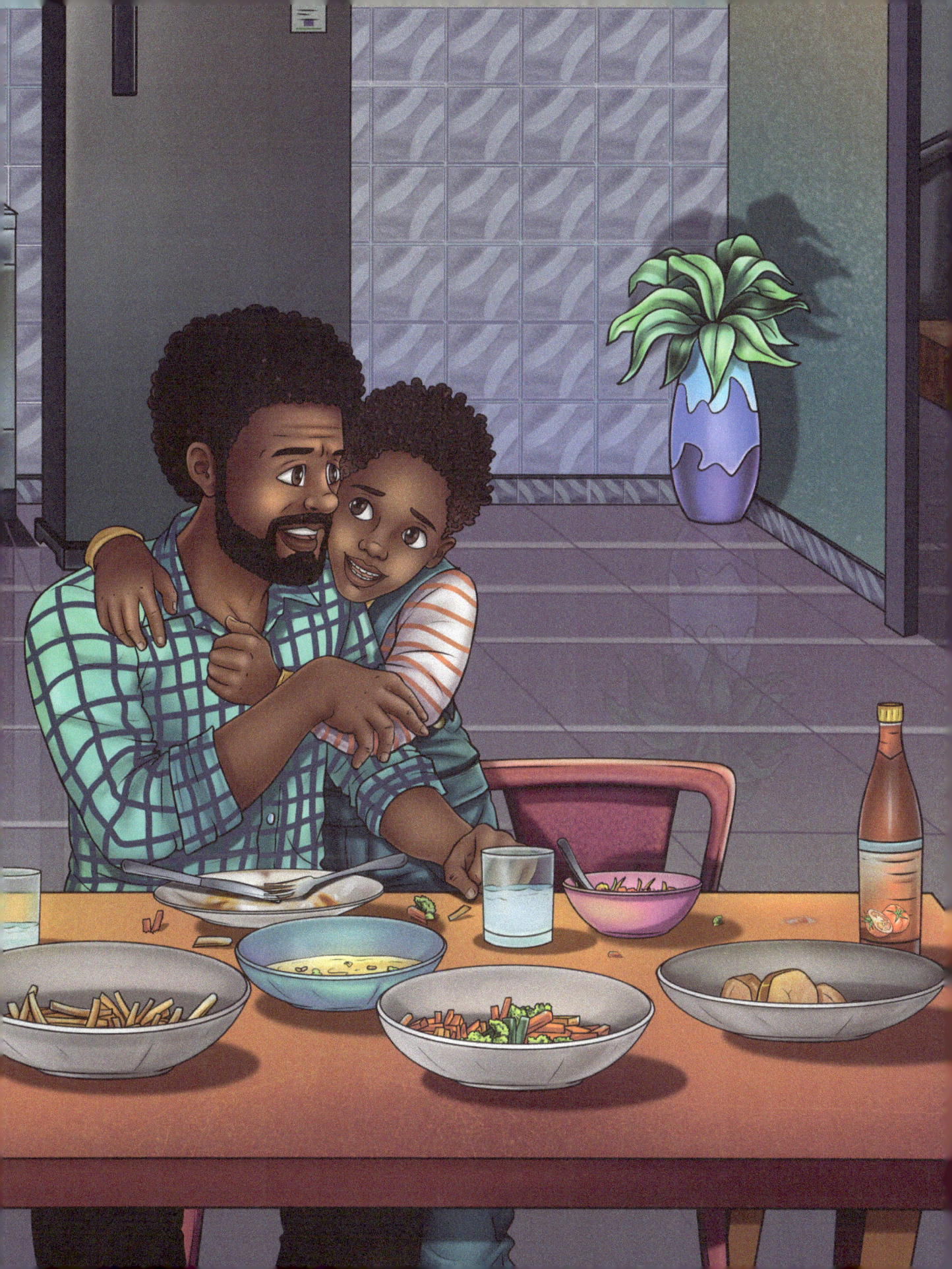

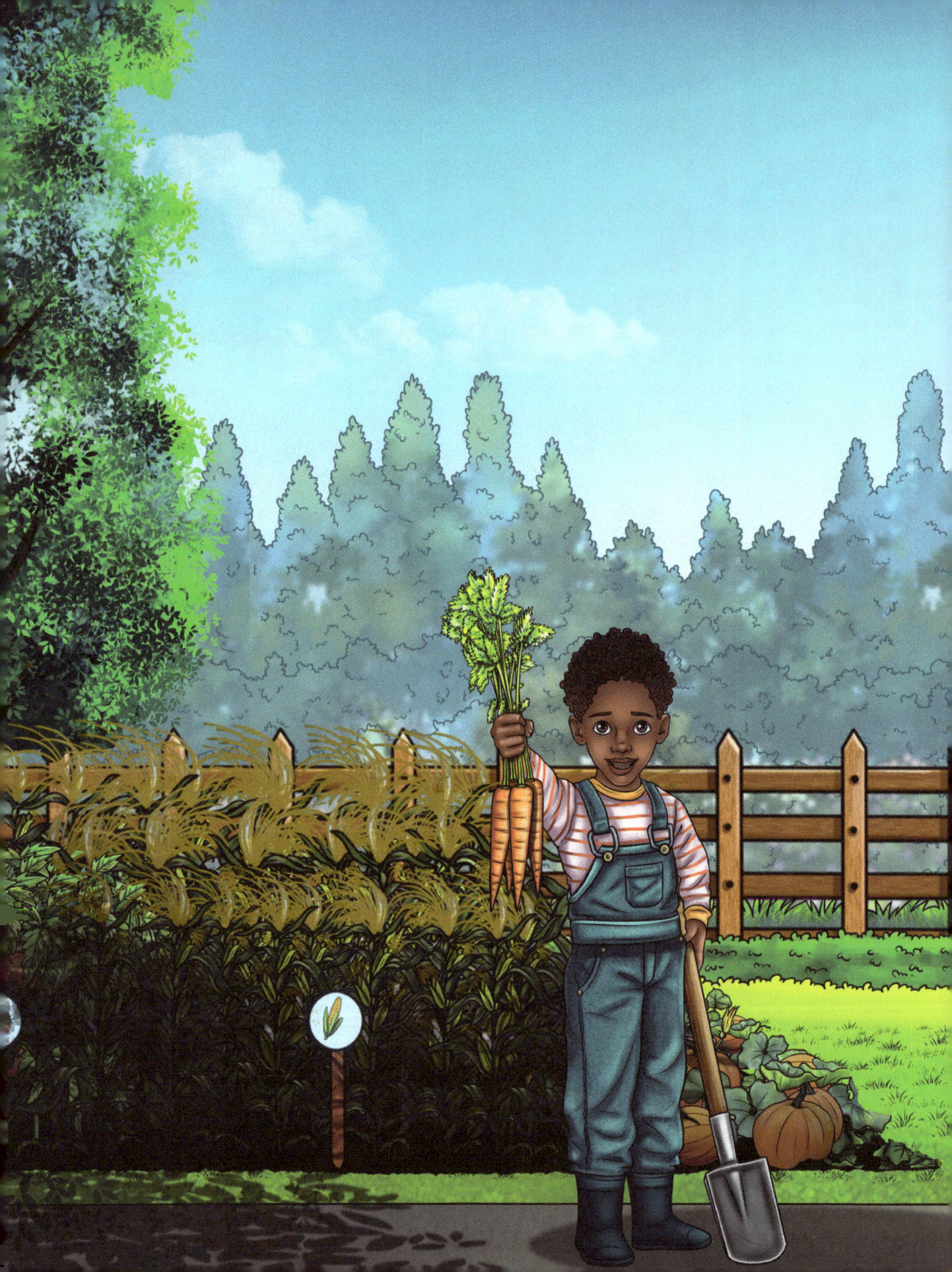

If you give a boy a garden, he'll become a gardener for life and want to teach others to be the same.

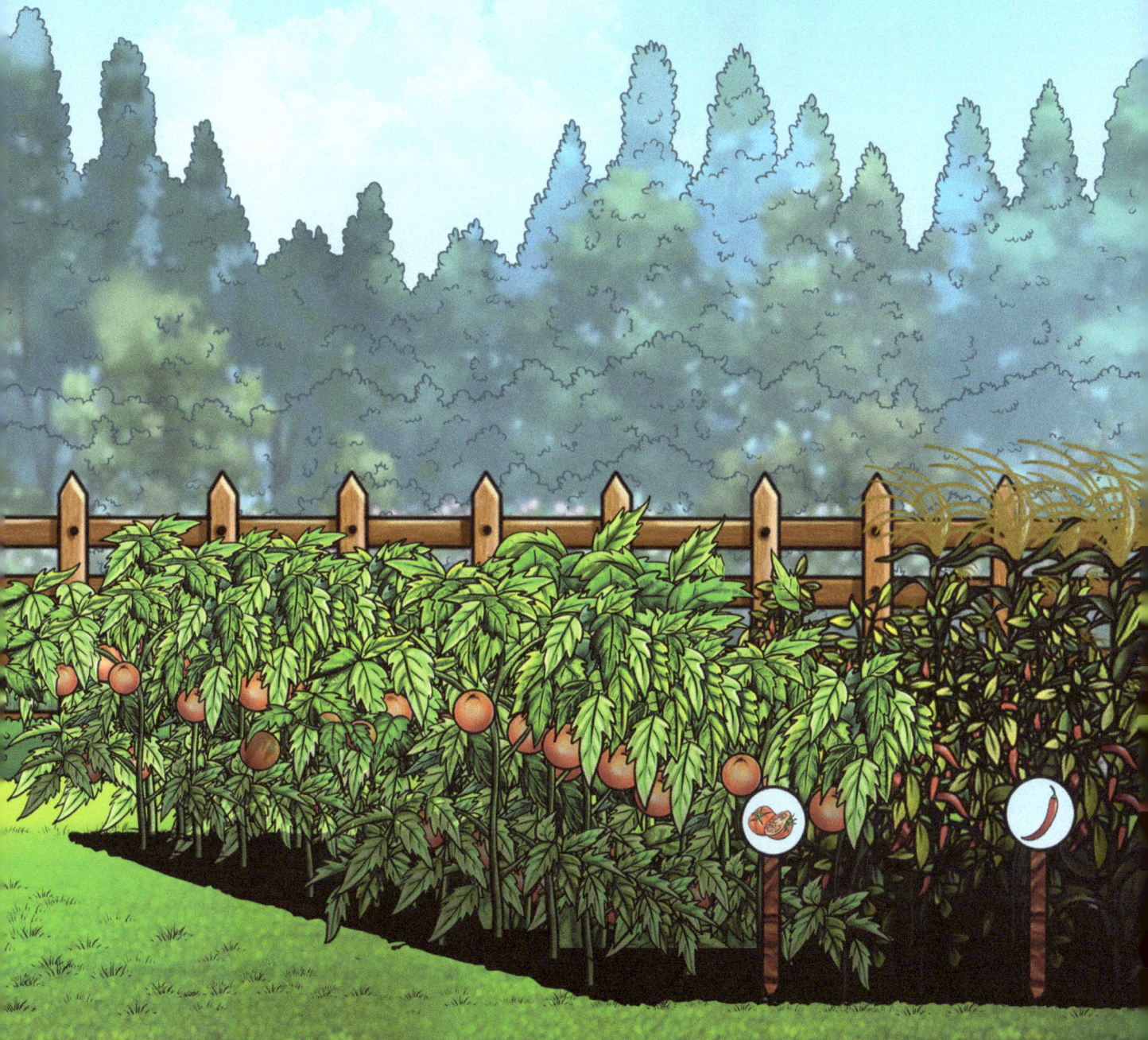

*To anyone who has ever planted a seed in a garden or life, give it your all, and it will produce a plentiful harvest. -DMJ*

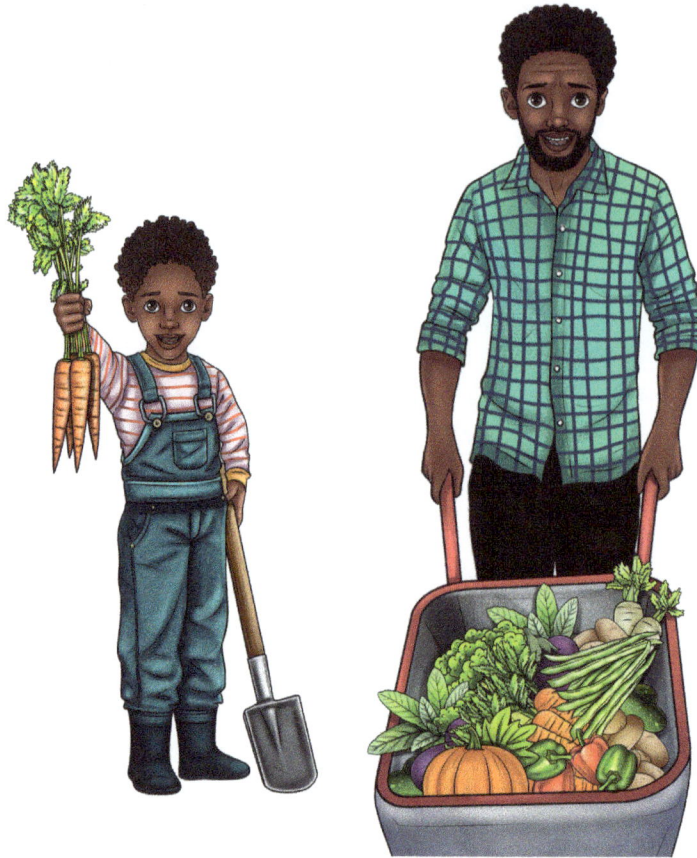

*If You Give a Boy a Garden*
*Copyright © 2022 by Hello Legendary Press LLC*
*Written by Danielle M. Jackson*
*Illustrated by Debasish Roy & Shivia Infotech Pvt.ltd*
*The illustrations in this book were created digitally.*
*Formatted by Mariana Cadavid Suarez*
*ISBN 978-1-7361-5668-1*
*Library of Congress Control Number: 2022901336*

www.ingramcontent.com/pod-product-compliance
Lightning Source LLC
Chambersburg PA
CBHW042351030426
42336CB00025B/3439